"We should see Melanie Klein's thought as an open work. It is a work that reinvents itself with each encounter with contemporary thought, fertilizing it and thus continuing to inspire new perspectives and sow new concepts derived from a deep understanding of her ideas. It is not a matter of accepting or rejecting her in its entirety, but of taking her ideas as a rich model of the functioning of the psychic apparatus. In her work, the process of acquiring knowledge has become a concept with metapsychological status and has been incorporated into most contemporary psychoanalytic theories."

Elisabeth da Rocha Barros and Elias Mallet da Rocha Barros, *training and supervising analysts and docents at the Brazilian Psychoanalytic Society of São Paulo (SBPSP); and fellows of the British Psychoanalytic Society and Institute*

I0092141

Why Read Klein? The Importance of Melanie Klein's work for Contemporary Psychoanalysis

Why Read Klein? explores the importance of Melanie Klein's work to contemporary psychoanalysis, her contributions as a key early psychoanalyst, and continued influence on contemporary psychoanalysts.

Klein's seminal work brought in several conceptual contributions that expanded psychoanalytic knowledge, sparking creativity and fostering a vibrant intellectual lineage. Her profound writings and enduring concepts embody a psychoanalytic legacy which has been constantly evolved and developed by various psychoanalysts who have drawn inspiration from her ideas over the years. This book presents the reverberations of her work in various authors, classic and contemporary. With an aim to encourage new forms of therapeutic action and conceptual understanding of her works, *Why Read Klein?* offers a modern interpretation of her ideas by incorporating films, poetry, and literary texts to illuminate her key concepts.

This book is essential reading for both practicing and in training psychoanalysts and psychotherapists seeking a comprehensive understanding of Klein's work and its relevance to contemporary clinical thought.

Elisa Maria de Ulhôa Cintra has a PhD in Clinical Psychology from Pontifícia Universidade Católica of São Paulo (PUC-SP). She is a psychoanalyst and is a professor on the Clinical Psychology Post-Graduate Studies Program at PUC-SP and the Faculty of Human and Health Sciences at PUC-SP. She is also the Coordinator of Laboratory at the Inter-Institutional Laboratory for Studies on Intersubjectivity and Contemporary Psychoanalysis (LIPSIC). In addition, she is the author of books and several articles published in specialized journals.

Marina F. R. Ribeiro, PhD, is a psychoanalyst, full professor and research supervisor and advisor for the Clinical Psychology Postgraduate Program at the University of São Paulo (USP). She is the Coordinator of Laboratory at the Inter-Institutional Laboratory for Studies on Intersubjectivity and Contemporary Psychoanalysis (LIPSIC). She is also the author of several books and papers and most recently co-authored *Reading Bion's Transformation* (2024) and edited *Why Read Ogden? The Importance of Thomas Ogden's Works for Contemporary Psychoanalysis* (2025).

Why Read Klein? The Importance of Melanie Klein's work for Contemporary Psychoanalysis

Edited by Elisa Maria de Ulhôa Cintra and Marina F. R. Ribeiro

Routledge
Taylor & Francis Group

LONDON AND NEW YORK

Designed cover image: © Marina F.R. Riberio

First English edition published 2026
by Routledge
4 Park Square, Milton Park, Abingdon, Oxon OX14 4RN

and by Routledge
605 Third Avenue, New York, NY 10158

Routledge is an imprint of the Taylor & Francis Group, an informa business

Authorised translation from the Spanish language edition, *Por que Klein?*, published by
Zagodoni Editora.

Trademark notice: Product or corporate names may be trademarks or registered trademarks,
and are used only for identification and explanation without intent to infringe.

British Library Cataloguing-in-Publication Data
A catalogue record for this book is available from the British Library

ISBN: 9781032950570 (hbk)
ISBN: 9781032947167 (pbk)
ISBN: 9781003583035 (ebk)

DOI: 10.4324/9781003583035

Typeset in Optima
by Newgen Publishing UK

To Melanie Klein, for her deeply sensitive clinical intuition and her remarkable courage as a pioneering psychoanalytic woman of her time.

Contents

x *Contents*

About the Authors

Elisa Maria de Ulhôa Cintra, has a PhD in Clinical Psychology from Pontifícia Universidade Católica of São Paulo (PUC-SP). She is a psychoanalyst and is a professor on the Clinical Psychology Post-Graduate Studies Program at PUC-SP and the Faculty of Human and Health Sciences at PUC-SP. She is also the Coordinator of Laboratory at the Inter-Institutional Laboratory for Studies on Intersubjectivity and Contemporary Psychoanalysis (LIPSIC). In addition, she is the author of books and several articles published in specialized journals.

Marina F. R. Ribeiro, PhD, is a psychoanalyst, full professor, and research supervisor and advisor for master's and PhD students in the Clinical Psychology Postgraduate Program at the University of São Paulo (USP). She is the Coordinator of Laboratory at the Inter-Institutional Laboratory for Studies on Intersubjectivity and Contemporary Psychoanalysis (LIPSIC). She is also the author of several books and papers and most recently co-authored *Reading Bion's Transformation* (2024) and edited *Why Read Ogden? The Importance of Thomas Ogden's Works for Contemporary Psychoanalysis* (2025).

Acknowledgments

Producing a book is always a collaborative endeavor, supported and encouraged by a network of contributors too numerous to name individually.

First and foremost, we express our profound gratitude to Daniel Kupermann and Adriano Zago for inviting us to contribute to this prestigious series in Portuguese, where we are privileged to be in such a distinguished company.

We deeply appreciate the creative freedom granted to us in presenting this text, which we believe enriches the body of literature about Melanie Klein. Our heartfelt thanks go to Luís Cláudio Figueiredo for the profound influence of his ideas, which resonate throughout the lines and interludes of this book, shaping it in immeasurable ways.

We are also sincerely grateful to Elizabeth Lima da Rocha Barros and Elias M. da Rocha Barros for their Prologue, which eloquently underscores the enduring impact of Melanie Klein's thinking on contemporary psychoanalysis.

This book also reflects our ongoing collaboration and shared dedication to teaching Melanie Klein's work at the Pontifical Catholic University of São Paulo (PUC-SP) and the University of São Paulo Institute of Psychology (IPUSP), as well as in undergraduate and graduate programs, fostering new generations of scholars both today and in the future.

We would like to extend our gratitude to the students and supervisees, whose direct or indirect contributions have been invaluable to this project. Additionally, we wish to thank the Department of Clinical Psychology at IPUSP for providing funding that supported part of the translation process.

Finally, we are grateful to Routledge for accepting this project for publication in English, ensuring this work reaches a broader international audience.

Foreword

Why read Klein today?

Elisa Maria de Ulhôa Cintra and
Marina F. R. Ribeiro

Why read Melanie Klein? And why today? These are the questions that illuminate this book. Thinking about the transmission of Klein's legacy leads directly to the effects that her writings have been producing and to the infinity of authors that have followed her around the world. It is, therefore, a seminal work, whose conceptions contain seeds of future thoughts, arousing, nourishing, and creating a living posterity.

There is no doubt that the reach of an author is measured in their posterity, in their ability to nourish thought and arouse new forms of therapeutic action and conceptual understandings. Driven by all this fecundity of Klein, we present, in this book, the reverberations of her work in various authors, classic and contemporary, in a way that is unique to our understanding and trajectory.

Following Klein's enlightenment project, and her proposal to come into contact with emotional experience, we could only write this book from our significant encounters with people and patients that we were fortunate to meet and who became our internal objects, in the slow incorporation of the lived experience. Without our internal objects, we cannot live. They are the ones who encourage us to turn to others, to deal with daily confrontations, to perform heroic feats, or leave us isolated and lost in our arrogance and omnipotence.

Internal objects – ours and those of our patients – give us a lot of work and make us seek an energetic balance, albeit always unstable, between the force of drives and the network of first symbolizations. Without them, the drive energy, being a blind force, tries to break through directly, through repetition, acting out, and enactments. A plot of objects with Enlightenment traits helps a lot when we are forced to fight with archaic internal objects, which remain active in the deep layers of our superego and can paralyze us.

Over time, Melanie Klein herself became for us an internal object of love and knowledge, encouraging us to work on omnipotence, arrogance, narcissism, the impossibility of mourning, of letting the past pass; finally, the core of madness that exists in each of us. The genius of her work is also assessed in these tiny and unconfessable effects, in the intimacy of each analysis and daily life, without disregarding the more visible effects in the immense pro-duction of her best-known followers. Among them are Bion and Winnicott, as well as many others who drank from Kleinian intuitions; later, French readers also joined them, such as Pontalis, Green, Roussillon, Florence Guignard. And we have, still, the English and American authors, like Rosenfeld, Searles, Grotstein, Ogden, Bollas, Britton, Casper, Hinshelwood, Symington, Steiner, in addition to two Italian Bionians: Bolognini and Antonino Ferro.

Among the French authors, Julia Kristeva[1], so linked to the works of Freud and Lacan, writes a book in which she celebrates the genius of Melanie Klein, highlighting the permeability to anguish that was hidden in an apparent security:

> The cohabitation with anxiety, symbolized, and therefore possible to live with, since it is elaborated through thought, gave her the taste and the strength not to retreat in the face of psychosis. ... [this reminds us that] freedom always strengthens through borderline experiences.
>
> (Kristeva, 1999, p. 21)

Klein, Kristeva highlights, did not dedicate herself to the political aspects of madness, but expanded her knowledge

> by discovering in the newborn a paranoid-schizoid ego, or by stating that 'the depressive position is indispensable for acquiring language', skillfully specifying 'the deep mechanisms that lead to the destruction of psychic space and the murder of the life of the spirit that threaten the modern era'.

> (...) through her, psychoanalysis has led us to the core of the human psyche to discover therein madness, which is both its driving force and its impasse. Melanie Klein's work is among those that have contributed most to our understanding of our being as it is a malaise, under its various aspects: schizophrenia, psychosis, depression, mania, autism, delays and inhibitions, catastrophic anxiety, fragmentation of the self, among others. And if it does not provide us with magical keys to avoid it, she helps us to provide optimal support and a chance for modulation towards a rebirth, perhaps.
>
> (Kristeva, 1999, p. 21)

The discomfort described above can be associated with the great social dis-comfort of the last one hundred and twenty years, and both can be linked to what Kristeva called the destruction of psychic space, thought by Klein, and the murder of the life of the spirit, thought by Hanna Arendt. For it was this destruction, we believe, that led to Nazi crimes, communist genocides, or racial genocides of the twentieth century, and that still leads to countless fundamentalisms of our historical moment.

The current discomfort comes from not being able to think, not being able to create a psychic space in which destructiveness and violence can take shelter and be lived on the symbolic plane, more than through impulsive and thoughtless acts. A place of contact, in which at least a part of the violence can transform into a desire to know and into works of culture, in the service of well-being. This was, after all, the enlightenment dream of Freud and Klein: to expand the psychic space.

And that is precisely what we seek in this book! With the intention of revealing the potency of Kleinian clinical thought, we have followed a different trajectory from so many others that have already been written, including the one produced by one of the authors along with Luís Cláudio Figueiredo: Melanie Klein: style and thought (2004).

At the same time that we present Kleinian concepts, we also indicate to the reader some of their expansions, bringing contemporary psychoanalysts who have studied Klein's work in depth into the dialogue, not necessarily being considered Kleinians.

To remember the capacity of Melanie Klein's work to disseminate and create new thoughts, we will refer, in particular, to three authors that we can consider as heirs of her lineage: Bion, Winnicott, and Ogden.

Another characteristic of this book is that we use films, books, poetry to reflect on the concepts, making the arduous theoretical presentation a little more playful, in the Winnicottian sense of the term, which considers playing an act of creation. In addition, some texts gathered here have already been previously published, in magazines and books by fellow psychoanalysts; others are based on our articles and books. We then collected the various references to Klein's work that mark our academic and clinical trajectory to offer the reader an unprecedented set built from our partnership.

Note

1 The translator has rendered all citations from Julia Kristeva freely.

References

Cintra, E. M. U. and Figueiredo, L. C. (2004). *Melanie Klein: Estilo e pensamento* (translation: Melanie Klein: style and thought) São Paulo: Escuta.

Kristeva, J. (1999). Le génie féminin: la vie, la folie, les mots: Hannah Arendt, Melanie Klein, Colette. Paris: Fayard. (translation: The Feminine Genius: Life, Madness, Words: Hannah Arendt, Melanie Klein, Colette).

Prologue

Melanie Klein yesterday, today, and tomorrow[1]

Elizabeth Lima da Rocha Barros and
Elias M. da Rocha Barros

Revolutions in thought, occurring in various fields of knowledge, are not always perceived at the moment they are outlined and developed[2].

We believe that in recent years there has been a rearrangement in the articulation of the basic concepts of psychoanalysis. An indication of this is the result of the survey conducted by the Editors/Coordinators of the International Encyclopedic Dictionary of Psychoanalysis, still in the elaboration phase, sponsored by the IPA (International Psychoanalytical Association). Among the five concepts considered most important for psychoanalytic clinical work – a survey conducted with about 400 authors, divided among the three continents – two were identified as distinctly Kleinian in origin: projective identification and containment, while the others, as one might expect, are unconscious, transference, and countertransference.

Recently, a colleague remarked that the number of citations of Melanie Klein in the bibliographies of papers published in São Paulo had dramatically decreased in recent years, expressing concern about the waning interest in this author. Many of the concepts developed by Melanie Klein are now directly incorporated into psychoanalysis or have become fertile ground for conceptual advancement, without necessarily acknowledging their origin.

Therefore, the research to assess the weight and importance of Klein in psychoanalysis should not only seek direct citations of her name but also examine the concepts originating from her work and those newly developed as a result of her thinking, such as expansions of the concept of projective identification, reverie, container, and the contained, among others.

This reflection leads us to consider: what defines a creative author is the introduction of a new issue that can no longer be ignored, thus constantly producing impacts that constitute new seeds for the advancement of thought.

From this perspective, our object of study would not be Melanie Klein as a historical figure associated with potentially outdated thinking, but rather the constitutive logic of her thought and its relevance today. It is essential to inquire: with which concepts did she approach certain clinical situations? And how did Klein articulate these concepts with clinical practice?

Another sign of this revolution in understanding psychoanalytic concepts is the attention given to both the construction of what we call the "Psychoanalytic Mind" and the construction and effects of language. Language is understood as a tool for creating experiences associated with "how it is" for the analyst to be with the patient and for the patient to be with the analyst. Both tendencies are influenced by theoretical–clinical currents inspired by Kleinian and Bionian thought.

We believe that Melanie Klein has gained autonomy in relation to her position within psychoanalytic thought; historically limited to the head of a School, she now integrates into the world of contemporary psychoanalytic ideas. Klein has freed herself from the limitation imposed by the adjective "Kleinian", which she always rejected, as she considered herself a follower of Freud rather than the head of a School. She was also the author who presented the most significant complement to Freud's theory of the human mind since the foundation of our discipline. Moreover, she generated a great deal of potentially enriching controversy, provided we are able to distance ourselves from ideological and doctrinal disputes. These dialogues about controversies continue to bear fruit.

From this angle, we should view Melanie Klein's thought as an open work. It is a work that reinvents itself with each encounter with contemporary thought, fertilizing it, and thus will continue to inspire new perspectives and sow new concepts derived from a profound understanding of her ideas. It is not a matter of accepting or rejecting her in its entirety, but of taking her work as a rich model of the functioning of the psychic apparatus.

Perhaps, instead of "legacy", we should approach her contribution not from the perspective of something that has been left to us, but rather as a living form of conception of the psychic apparatus that continues to have effects on current psychoanalytic thought. Her legacy is not delimited, nor has her thinking reached its final form. We should read it as a still-living thought that integrates into contemporary psychoanalysis, and for this reason, we continue to study her today! Klein did not construct the final version of her work, even though her life ended, as it continues to produce living effects and, in doing so, also transforms itself. This dialectical perspective is crucial to preserve when approaching and studying the work of Melanie Klein.

Recently, a message circulated on internet social networks with a photo of Melanie Klein accompanied by a thought attributed to her. The text read: "Whoever eats from the fruit of knowledge is expelled from some paradise". This post is emblematic of what we think. The paradise from which the knowledgeable individual is expelled refers to the liberation from a false security based on a state of mind that prioritizes superficiality and emotional detachment in human relationships, sustained by idealizations. Ceasing to be superficial, through the refinement of our capacity for reflection, being profound and responsible in our interpersonal relationships becomes a factor of mental health, in the conception of psychoanalysis that we practice today, and this premise derives directly from Klein's work. Being able to maintain intimate

emotional relationships is essential as a factor of maturity. Human development in our author's conception is not linear but dialectical, and closer to a
spiral process. Mental health, from Klein's perspective, is always threatened
in its stability and thus must be permanently regained. Mental well-being
or balance is not the natural consequence of successful and somewhat pre-
programmed development. Mental health can be accompanied by a feeling
of loneliness, resulting from the realization that there is no idealized state of
perfect integration, which existed or was unconsciously fantasized about in a
pre-verbal phase of fusion or near-fusion with the mother. Integration involves
abandoning idealizations, both of external objects and aspects of the self. The
well-internalized object is not confused with perfection.

In her work, the process of acquiring knowledge has become a concept
with metapsychological status and has been incorporated into most contemporary psychoanalytic theories.

It's important to consider that even texts considered classics acquire new
connotations as they are read over the years. It is common for a recent text
to shed new light on classic articles. Texts undergo transformations through
what Octavio Paz (1975) called intertextuality. Texts from different eras
interact with each other, producing new meanings or simultaneously erasing
meanings that have become anachronistic.

The new idea that leads to an original perspective is the product of a re-
examination of traditions in dialectical confrontation with the present. Texts,
in this case, are not just the written ones; they also include discussions and
their reverberations within a particular culture, whether institutional or not.

Thus, delving into the understanding of Klein's work is a way to deepen our
understanding of psychoanalysis itself through knowledge of the sources that
inspire the movement of ideas in our field.

Reading Klein's texts requires a great commitment from the reader, who
needs time to study them, to be able to separate what is a clinical observation
from what is a theoretical speculation, full of consequences.

Klein developed her psychoanalytic vocation driven by the desire to
understand the mechanisms of inhibition that prevent a child from fully
developing their emotional and cognitive capacities. She gradually discovers
that this child is a victim of tyranny imposed by their unconscious destructive phantasies that prevent them from exercising their curiosity about the
world of things and people, including themselves. Fear is the basis of tyranny,
generating a coercive psychic reality based on the law of retaliation and the
violence of the death drive. Only the liberation of our capacity to love, based
on the understanding of the logic underlying our unconscious phantasies, can
free us and allow the full flourishing of our affective and intellectual capacities. In the beginning of her inquiries, we find the roots of her conception of
what she called the epistemophilic instinct and later, the drive to know. This
idea later gave rise to the proposal of the links K-K in Bion's work.

Pascal said that instincts are the reasons of the heart about which reason
knows nothing. Klein seeks to decipher these reasons of the heart through

understanding the sense and meaning of what she characterizes as unconscious phantasies. Phantasies are derived and, at the same time, organizers of emotional experiences, which constitute cores generating meaning that, in turn, color our emotions and interfere with our perceptions. Unconscious phantasy is, above all, an active mode of unconscious thinking that acquires a certain stability, generating meanings that cluster around a core meaning-giver, which operates as an organizer of psychic life and thus creates links with other emotional experiences. Traumatic unconscious phantasies shape a lived situation that was initially incomprehensible and intolerable. However, by constituting itself as a core of meanings in psychic life, it also distorts other associated emotional experiences, becoming, despite its dynamism, a potentially distorting mode of attributing meaning to other emotional experiences. In some traumatic circumstances, an unconscious phantasy can freeze psychic life.

In Klein, emotions come to be considered in psychic structure as something comparable to connective tissue, operating as links between the various levels of psychic instances and corresponding experiences. It is Bion, once again, one of the most creative continuators of Kleinian thought, who will develop this aspect with great richness in studying attacks on these binding links.

For Melanie Klein and her followers, people suffer not only due to deficiencies, traumas, or repressions. They also suffer from a lack of emotional experiences that foster growth. From this perspective, it is not enough for psychoanalysis to be effective in uncovering repressions that prevent certain thoughts or feelings from coming to light, or to provide a facilitating environment that allows for the repair of past deficiencies. The presence of splitting and projective identification points to a fragmented mind, in which the various psychic instances do not communicate, and which has its capacity to symbolize impaired. This limitation in the ability to create symbols and, therefore, to think about emotions in a richer way, creates an internal atmosphere of emptiness, of lack of meaning for life. Under these conditions, certain thoughts never even get formulated.

In Klein, emotional "emptiness" does not equate to a blank slate. Instead of an emotional "blank", we have this psychic space filled with a negative, life-denying force. It is a negativizing zero. One of the legacies of this conception will be developed and greatly expanded by Bion (negative and negativizing emotions), Rosenfeld, and André Green (the force of the negative, also inspired by Hegel) when dealing with narcissism.

For Melanie Klein, reason itself and the principle of reality do not exist in a vacuum; they come from somewhere. And thus, they are also subject not only to conflicts and blockages but also mainly result from a deficiency in the capacity to construct an apparatus for thinking. To the amplified model that included not only defense mechanisms to eliminate anxiety-generating contents from consciousness, Klein adds the possibility of the ego itself and its internal objects splitting; in the same way that mental functions can be eliminated by this same process.

One of the implications of her observations and hypotheses is that personality is constituted of various levels that operate concomitantly, sometimes in harmony and consonance, and sometimes in open conflict. Thus, infantile aspects of personality operate simultaneously with adult aspects, sometimes dominating the personality, co-opting the adult into a mental functioning of an infantile nature, and sometimes integrating into adult functioning. These diverse instances with their own logics may or may not be in communication with each other and with the external world. Implicit in this approach is the differentiation between the historical child and the infantile (the infans) as a psychic instance. These ideas will later be deepened by Bion, Britton, Steiner, Meltzer, Rosenfeld, and Ferro, among others.

Bion used the metaphor of the midwife of the mind to refer to the analyst's function, just as the mother performs this function in emotionally caring for the baby, to the extent that she is able to, through the function of reverie, internalize and digest the emotional experiences that are intolerable for the baby. It could also be added that this perspective generates the idea that the session is an incubator of new symbolic forms.

When working oriented by a hypothetical concept of normality, our model of pathology will be based on an assessment of the cost that the individual pays for resisting the assimilation of new experiences. And, in this way, one condemns oneself to an emotional superficiality that manifests itself in the way one relates to people and the world in general. This may be one of Melanie Klein's central theses.

We would like to emphasize the importance of the concept of positions in understanding the processes of subjectivity formation. The concept of positions was introduced by Klein, and its study was greatly expanded, especially by authors such as Thomas Ogden (1994, 1997, 2011), John Steiner (2017), and Ronald Britton (1998).

Positions are, above all, ways of generating and organizing experience and of relating to affects according to the predominant anxiety. These operate through a continuous oscillation of a dialectical nature and following a certain spiral movement. One position exists in relation to the other. The first of these, the paranoid-schizoid, has as its basic modus operandi a dynamic based on the need to rid oneself of excess anxiety through a violent cutting off from it. It defends itself from persecutory anxiety by splitting, projecting, denying emotions. Under the auspices of its functioning, experiences are decontextualized and therefore become ahistorical (exist outside of time), the various networks of affects that constitute us are disconnected from each other, the capacity to create symbols is impoverished, and the expressive aspects of experience lose strength.

In turn, the depressive position aims to integrate sometimes contradictory affects through a process of elaboration that involves producing symbols capable of containing emotional experiences through thought. It situates experiences in a historical context and expands their meanings through the connection of affective networks. Ronald Britton seminally amplifies the consequences of the permanent and dialectical interaction of these two positions. He associates this dialectic with a complex process of progressive development of the capacity for interactive integration that leads to moments of progression and regression, although they never return exactly to the previous plane.

Another important concept, with several ramifications, in Klein's work is that of projective identification. For us, a central point present in the notion of projective identification lies in the fact that it, through the processes that constitute it, involves choices and intense negotiations between subject and object, both at the intrapsychic and intersubjective levels. These negotiations are far from following a unidirectional logic. Projective identification modifies the identity and perception of the agents involved and is directly related to the constitution of the identity of both elements of the dyad and, particularly, how this identity is experienced. The question, in this case, is when the subject is the subject of their feelings and develops what Ogden (1994, 1997, 2011) called I-ness, or when they are lived by their feelings, constituting an experience in me-ness, to use the terminology from Ogden (1994, 1997, 2011) himself. The issue involved is the position of the Ego in the experience, whether it lives it actively or passively. And in this context, the operation of projective identification is central, as it deprives the subject of their "I-ness".

I would also like to emphasize, as Susanna Goretti (2007) does, that the introduction of the concept of projective identification has modified psychoanalysis as a whole, even though these modifications are not explicitly attributed to the introduction of this term. As García Marques (2008) says: Ideas are not anyone's. They fly around like angels.

Klein (1946), by suggesting that the patient projects into the analyst's mind and not onto it, introduces the idea that the patient does something with the analyst's mind, whether in reality or in fantasy, and in this process induces feelings associated with an invitation to action, either for the analyst to feel certain feelings or to engage in the performance of a certain role. In a way, we could say that the one who projects infects the other with a new identity. Implicit here, among other things, is the concept of enactment, also central to our current reflections. From this statement arises the progressive incorporation into prevailing psychoanalytic ideas that a good part of the movements in the session can only be understood as intersubjective phenomena. Roosevelt Cassorla (2015), among Brazilian psychoanalysts, has developed these ideas with great mastery.

This proposition has a direct impact on how countertransference comes to be viewed from a clinical standpoint. In the history of psychoanalytic concepts, we could say that initially countertransference could be seen as analogous to a photograph of a relational moment. Subsequently, with the evolution of the understanding of the analytic relationship as an inter-relational (bipersonal) process, countertransference came to be analogically compared to a film, something that results from the movement of many photographs (Ferro, 1995,

1999). From this moment on, we can no longer speak of countertransference in isolation and we begin to associate it with what Bion called reverie (Rocha Barros & Rocha Barros, 2016). At this moment, the ongoing mental processes in the analyst's mind became the focus of investigation and the field from which interpretation is elaborated. From this underlying implication arises the entire work of Bion, Ogden, Britton, among others.

It is interesting to note how the concept of projective identification accounts for certain phenomena described by the great novelists of our time. Balzac, for example, observes: Vice asks for nothing, it offers everything.

This observation by a character in Balzac touches on one of the central aspects of the concept as we use it today; namely, how a person, through words, or even without using them, leads the other to feel certain feelings, alters their perception, induces roles, and thus invites the members of the interacting dyad to behave according to a pattern that is not their own, or rather, saying that it is and is not their pattern. Projective identification simultaneously affirms and denies the subject. In this way, through projective identifications, the subject ceases to be a subject and shapes the world according to their biased needs.

One of the problems involved in the phenomena described under the term projective identification focuses on how it is transmitted to the other, either in the form of feelings or in the induction of roles, as a discursive or representational-imaginary symbol. In this context, when Bion and Rosenfeld refer to the communicative aspect of projective identification, we are thinking of something more than that encompassed by the term informing. Projective identification does more than inform about a state of mind, as we have already mentioned in previous paragraphs; it is closer to the idea of inoculating, infusing than informing; hence the role of evocation and expressiveness in symbolic constitution processes.

To better understand this issue, let's refer to the phenomenon of expressiveness as described in the philosophy of art. This term, as we are using it now, initially referred to an aspect of art that aimed not only to describe or represent emotions but centrally to transmit them, producing them in the other or in oneself from an evocation, a mental representation colored by emotion. Expressiveness precedes communicative capacity through words.

Evocation is a form of non-discursive expression. Although it is mostly permeated by the patient's verbalizations and, as a consequence, allowing other connections than those of discursive logic to appear, mediated by words, thus expanding the forms of representations of affective relations.

Evocations often take on imagistic[3] forms, which we propose are equally representative of the feelings involved in the living relationship of that moment, and which we assume to be expressive of the relationship with others and with the world. In the Kleinian perspective, we are talking about projective identifications that Bion, in turn, considered to be a form of preverbal thought, a primitive matrix of ideograms.

To conclude, we revisit the words published on the internet, mentioned above: "Whoever eats from the fruit of knowledge is expelled from some paradise". Words that speak exactly of this encounter and disconnection and again encounter of knowledge that drives us towards maintaining an attitude of curiosity and vitality in the daily exercise of our professional activity. We also emphasize that studying the constitutive dynamics of Melanie Klein's work helps us understand the internal mechanisms that govern the processes of conceptual expansion of psychoanalysis itself.

Kristeva (1978, 2004) asserts: Every text is constructed as a mosaic of quotations; every text is absorption and transformation of another text[4]. If texts are studied from this point of view, we may conclude, for example, that a concept as contemporary as reverie was already seeded in Freud's work in the notion of equally floating attention, although at that time still isolated from an intersubjective relationship. From this angle, the issue of reverie and intersubjectivity (so contemporary!) was prominently present in the concept of projective identification introduced by Klein. In other words, it is impossible to understand the importance of intersubjectivity without knowing its relationship with the problematic of projective identification, a term that contains immense complexity within it.

It is only when we expand our capacity to communicate with ourselves (and consequently also with others), through the permanent creation of new symbols – the basis of thought construction – that we develop the ability to deal with psychic suffering and create the conditions for a deeper understanding of the human world around us. From this perspective, it is through psychic truth that the patient discovers about themselves, and that previously they were unable to think or feel, and therefore unable to put into words, that the individual becomes able to live the life that previously remained unlived, to use an expression dear to Winnicott.

We believe we have highlighted, even if briefly, some of the most relevant contributions in Melanie Klein's work and her influence on psychoanalysis yesterday, today, and tomorrow.

Notes

1 Yesterday, today, and tomorrow is also the name of an inaugural lecture given by Hanna Segal in November 2001 at the Institute of Psychoanalysis in London and published on the Melanie Klein Trust website <www.melanie-klein-trust.org.uk>.

2 This prologue is based on some recent joint work of mine and Elizabeth's, especially on conferences presented in 2017. After so many years of collaborative work, it is difficult today to separate what is my contribution from what is Elizabeth's.

3 We are using the word "image" in the same sense as Susanne Langer (1967) does, namely, as roughly defined as a material of the imagination (p. 59).

4 NT: Translator's rendition.

References

Britton, R. (1998). *Belief and imagination: Explorations in psychoanalysis*. London, England: Routledge.

Cassorla, R. M. S. (2015). *O psicanalista, o teatro dos sonhos e a clínica do enactment*. London: Karnac. (translation: The psychoanalyst, the theater of dreams, and the clinic of enactment).

Cassorla, R. M. S. (2018). *The psychoanalyst, the theater of dreams and the clinic of enactment*. Routledge.

Ferro, A. (1995). *La tecnica nella psicoanalisi infantile: Il bambino, l'analista, il campo emotivo*. Torino, Italy: Bollati Boringhieri. (translation: Technique in child psychoanalysis: The child, the analyst, the emotional field).

Ferro, A. (1999). *The bi-personal field: Experiences in child analysis*. Philadelphia: Psychology Press.

Goretti, G. (2007). Projective identification: A theoretical investigation of the concept starting from "Notes on some schizoid mechanisms". *International Journal of Psychoanalysis, 88*(2), 387–405.

Klein, M. (1946/1975). Notes on some schizoid mechanism. In: *Envy and gratitude and other works*. New York: The Free Press.

Kristeva, J. (1978). *Semiótica* – Vol. I. Fundamentos. (Free translation: Semiotics).

Kristeva, J. (2004). *Female genius. v. 2. Melanie Klein*. 304 pp. Columbia University Press. (Original work published in 2002).

Langer, S. (1967,1982). *Mind: An essay on human feeling*. Johns Hopkins University Press.

Marques, G. (2008). *Of love and other demons*. Vintage. (Original work published in 1994).

Ogden, T. (1994). *Subjects of analysis*. Northvale, Janson Aronson and Karnak.

Ogden, T. (1997). *Revêrie and interpretation*. Jason Aronson

Ogden, T. (2011). Reading Susan Isaacs: Toward a radical revised theory of thinking. *International Journal of Psychoanalysis, 92*(4), 925–942.

Paz, O. (1975). *The children of the mire*. (R. Phillips, Trans.). Harvard University Press.

Petot, J.M. (1990). *Melanie Klein*. Vol. 1. (C. Trollope, Trans.). International Universities Press.

Petot, J.M. (1990). *Melanie Klein*. Vol. 2. (C. Trollope, Trans.). International Universities Press.

Rocha Barros, E., & Rocha Barros, E. (2016). The function of evocation in the working-through of the countertransference; projective identification, reverie, and the expressive function of the mind-Reflections inspired by Bion's work. In Levite, H; Civitarese, G (Ed.) *The W. R. Bion tradition*. Karnak.

Rolland, J.C. (2006). *Avant d'être celui qui parle*. Gallimard.

Steiner, J. (2017). Introduction, outline and critical review of Klein's lectures and seminars on technique. In *Lecturers on technique by Melanie Klein*. Routledge.

Introduction

Elisa Maria de Ulhôa Cintra and Marina F. R. Ribeiro

Melanie Klein brought us several conceptual contributions that expanded psychoanalytic knowledge, such as the notion of internal objects and that object relations are present from the beginning of life. She never abandoned the idea of a conflict between life and death drives, as described by Freud, nor the dimension of intensities, that is, the economic vertex. However, by emphasizing the universe of objects and phantasy scenarios, she expanded the dynamic understanding of the psyche, postulating that all aspects of psychic functioning are linked to internal and external objects in constant transformation.

The initial object relations are understood by Klein as ambivalent; love and hate present themselves from the beginning and mark the experience with the internal and external world. The beginning of life is, therefore, a chaotic emotional experience, with moments in which sadism predominates, which is the purest expression of the intensity and violent character of the demands for love and attention. It is the time of oscillations between everything and nothing, of insatiable desires for love and destruction, of the demand for the permanence of the other by our side, or of radical withdrawal of this other who hurt us.

Without rest, Klein directs our gaze and makes us sensitive to the tragic aspects of human existence: love, hate, losses, anxieties, boredom, compassion, death, fatigue, condemnatory judgments, persecutory thoughts, rejection and, finally, envy and its deadly strategies to destroy the value of everything that life has offered us.

Indeed, perhaps the first question that draws our attention in the clinical work of our author is her ability to stay close to the experience of suffering and the anguish of patients. With anguish, we reach the most basic ground of psychic functioning, we touch what is most visceral, most intimate, most deeply determinant of all psychic organization. Melanie Klein believed this to be the most "crucial" conductor of analytical listening, which best leads to the infrastructure of psychic happening. The hypothesis is that by listening and intervening in the register of anguish we reach the level of the forces that generate psychotic suffering and produce neurosis, in its unconscious and

DOI: 10.4324/9781003583035-1

inaccessible dimension; to approach this nucleus, however, it is essential to have a sensitive listening, the Einfühlung, of which Freud and Ferenczi speak.

We can affirm, moreover, that without empathic resonance – Einfühlung – with the patient's suffering it is not possible to conduct an analysis. Melanie Klein deeply appropriates this empathy in her analytical listening, being therefore an heir of Ferenczi in this aspect. On the other hand, it is possible to say that the psychic apparatus in Freud, Abraham, and Klein is predominantly intrapsychic; whereas in Ferenczi and in the heirs of Klein – Bion, Winnicott and contemporary psychoanalysts, the psyche begins to be thought of in an intersubjective way; that is, constituting itself in the plot of relations with other psychic subjects, without ever leaving aside the intrapsychic dimension.

What can be affirmed with certainty about the Kleinian legacy is that the author's emphasis on the notions of introjection and projection, and the developments of the concept of projective identification, allowed a clearer perception of the importance of the analyst coming into contact with the patient's feelings and thoughts, to personally feel what is happening with him. In this tradition, the maternal and analytical functions of receiving, containing, elaborating and returning, digesting the primitive contents of the child and the patient – the reverie – became the basis of the most important transformations in analytical techniques in recent decades. And it was these modifications that allowed the analysis of children, psychotics, and other disturbances of the narcissistic axis, such as melancholy and some depressions.

Klein built the entire edifice of her work from the creation of a true clinical thought. And although we cannot place her in the lineage of intersubjectivity, her theory of projective identification, as it was being appropriated by her heirs, became, alongside Ferenczi's contributions, the matrix of the notion of countertransference, as understood by Paula Heimann, of future notions of field, theories of the analytical situation, and the third analytical.

Technical innovations of Klein and their reverberations in classic and contemporary authors

It is important to highlight that to treat psychosis and borderline cases, when the patient's ability to freely associate is not fluent, or even impossible, and for having cared for children from the beginning, Klein had to invent techniques that made possible a psychoanalytic listening where the analyst needs to practically create, with the patient, associative paths and trails, when these are absent or precariously constituted. She then dared to make the symbolic grafts necessary for work with the most difficult cases, like that of Dick.

It is from Klein that Bion thought about the need to give containment to the expressions of the patients, qualifying this attitude, this mental operation, through the notion of reverie, incorporated into a large part of current psychoanalytic practices.

The task of opening new paths to access the word and the narration of a story is, undoubtedly, a merit of Melanie Klein; certainly, the first psychoanalyst to practice, intuitively, the reverie or the ability to dream (dreaming) to refer to the unconscious psychic work that needs to be done on the emotional experience. More evidently than Freud, Klein drew attention to the overwhelming emotional experience, to the anguishes and archaic fears that can be gathered under the name of annihilation anxieties, which are so difficult to elaborate that it is impossible to do it alone.

Ogden, in turn, intensely rereading Bion's work, rediscovers in it four underlying principles to Bionian thought. Let us then see how it is possible to discern the Kleinian inheritance in each of them:

1. Thought is driven by the human need to know the truth, the reality of who we are and what is happening in our life.
2. The presence of two minds is necessary to think about a person's most disturbing thoughts.
3. The ability to think is developed so that a person can reconcile with thoughts that arise from their disturbing emotional experience.
4. There is, inherent to the personality, a psychoanalytic function: dreaming – or reverie – this is the main process through which this function manifests itself. (Ogden, 2009, p. 91)[1].

Regarding the first item, there is no doubt that the human need to know the truth relates to the enlightenment aspiration we spoke of earlier and that marked Klein's entire life, both in relation to herself and her patients. This can be verified from the beginning of her work, from her first case, the little Fritz, when she upheld the importance of the epistemophilic drive (Klein, 1923) that was inhibited in him – later, it was discovered that it was, in fact, her youngest son.

From the repression of the desire to know more about the origin of babies and the father's participation in the origin of life, Fritz had built a series of intellectual and affective inhibitions that were preventing him from continuing his development. Klein demonstrates, with this case, that it is always possible to shed the light of reason and empathetic understanding on the darkest aspects of the psyche, in order to lessen the weight of prejudices and moral judgments. These are not guided by the desire to know the most hostile aspects of reality, the deep roots of violence, and the most primitive practices of dominating others, such as conflicts and wars.

In relation to the other items listed by Ogden (2004), we would say that when one cannot think for oneself about the disturbing emotional experience, the subject needs the help of another person to dream "undreamt dreams and interrupted cries" (Ogden, 2004, p. 17). A person who cannot narrate themselves and is at the center of a movement of "letting oneself be spoken by others", in a way, "does not exist". It is tragic and radical to say this. It reminds us of the feeling of some patients who are numb and need to be vitalized and awakened. They need to get out of a state where they are inhabited by foreign voices and eyes, by hauntings that prevent them from having their own mind. They have not yet entered historical time and can only repeat what they have heard. The continuous and systematic work to engender and transform depressive positions is what leads to entering historical time, to the position of becoming a narrator: one who brings together past, present, and future, escaping from the imaginary capture about oneself. Many find themselves locked in a fixed idea about themselves, in the prison of not being able to think outside of a cocoon of images and representations that have frozen.

In the case of the analytic situation, it is the analyst who may initiate what Ogden referred to as an apparently non-analytic conversation. Thus, while attending, and being guided by his reverie, Ogden dares to free himself to subjects that are apparently outside the strict analysis of mental functioning and begins to talk with some patients about books or works of art. This apparently non-analytic conversation will function as a placenta; it will be the matrix of the future free association that was trapped in defenses, and from this strategy, the patient is released to enter into a classical analytic process. In these conversations, primary and secondary processes blend, allowing the installation of the patient's capacity to daydream, speaking-as-if-they-were-dreaming. On the analyst's side, these reveries bring understanding and insight into what is happening in the transference and the patient's other relationships.

Access to reverie is experienced by some patients as an awakening, a true birth to another emotional experience; only then do they become able to narrate their own lives and engage in the game of free association. "A life that is not narrated does not exist" – said the Portuguese writer, Lobo Antunes. It is a compelling idea.

Another example of the remarkable fruition of seeds of Kleinian thought is found in Ogden's book *Subjects of Psychoanalysis* (1994). The author considers the paranoid-schizoid and depressive positions as different ways of attributing meaning to emotional experience, which is different from saying that there are two ways of functioning, as proposed by Klein, and saying that there are two ways of giving meaning to existence: one that is paranoid-schizoid, and the other that is depressive.

The expansion of thought lies precisely in these small shifts of meaning. Ogden (1994) makes another shift, stating, more explicitly than Klein, that these two forms do not exist separately but in a dialectical relationship with each other. He then brings the Hegelian notion of dialectics into Melanie Klein's intuition as a strategy to broaden the original, to make it work in a new way.

The author also highlights that each of the ways of making sense of existence requires the other, and that they oscillate in the same way that, for Freud, the conscious mind only makes sense in relation to the unconscious mind; both do not exist separately. "The Kleinian subject" – Ogden asserts (1994, p. 34) – "exists not in any given position or hierarchical layering of positions, but in the dialectical tension created between positions". From this, we can infer that the place of the subject in psychoanalysis is a place in temporal movement, and it can be better understood by affirming that the psychic subject is a relation between two places, between two different ways of making sense of experience. In this perspective:

> The paranoid-schizoid position represents a psychological organization generating a state of being that is ahistorical, relatively devoid of the experience of an interpreting subject mediating between the sense of I-ness and one's lived sensory experience. This paranoid-schizoid mode contributes to the sense of immediacy and intensity of experience.
>
> (Ogden, 1994, p. 35)

On the other hand, the depressive position creates a subject who narrates themselves, capable of interpreting lived experiences and mediating between themselves and sensory experience, which allows entry into historical time, accessing past and future. The depressive position enables recognizing others as total and independent subjects, with an internal life similar to our own, giving rise to the ability to care for others, feel guilt, and make non-magical reparations for harm done in imagination and reality, increasing tolerance for pain and frustration; ultimately, generating a quality of life that possesses a richness of symbolic meanings.

Indeed, following Klein's intuition regarding the constant oscillation between the two positions, Ogden (1994) situates the subject between successive processes of splitting and integration, thereby constituting because it oscillates between positions, because it is temporalized; its process of constitution makes it a subject in perpetual wandering, in transition, a being in becoming.

It is inevitable to think that this reading of Klein is a creative way of using her discovery. Revisiting the last point mentioned, Ogden (1994) defamiliarizes us by saying that the depressive position, with its historicity and capacity to create symbols, should not be thought of as the quintessential place of the subject in Kleinian theory, just as the unconscious is not the place of the Freudian subject, as some think. In Freud and in Klein, the psychoanalytic subject is always nomadic, perpetually in transit between conscious and unconscious, between the paranoid-schizoid and depressive pole, in the "space (tension) created by the dialectical interplay of the different dimensions of experience" (Ogden, 1994, p. 48).

Another field in which Klein's thought bore fruit concerns the phenomenon of projective identification and countertransference. Before her, the analyst focused on the patient's psychic life; but, based on her theorizations, there began to be more consideration of the analyst's mental functioning, through their reverie, and their participation during the session.

The idea that everything the analyst thinks and feels is part of the transference inspired several authors who have been dedicated to the conception of the analytic field, generated by the patient–analyst dyad. It is worth mentioning here the Baranger couple, who, in the early 1960s, published a text about the analytic situation that became a classic, leading us to recognize the need, as analysts, to listen to ourselves more and to become more deeply involved in the analytic process.

For the Baranger couple (2008/1961–1962), projective and introjective identifications are exchanged between analyst and analysand, eliciting shared unconscious phantasies that facilitate or hinder the analytic process. From this perspective, negative therapeutic reaction becomes more intense when shared resistances, difficult to dissolve – the so-called bulwarks – are formed in a joint production of analyst and patient[2].

The next reference we bring to exemplify the importance of Klein's legacy and the fecundity of her thought is a clinical case by Winnicott (1977), where the precedence of Klein's insights is clearly seen, making it possible to understand the acute suffering of a two-year-old girl, named Piggle. The parents were therapists and were distressed, trying to understand what was happening with their daughter; however, due to the impossibility of attending a classic five-session weekly therapy, as they lived outside London, the child's condition was described through letters addressed to Winnicott.

Piggle's treatment took place about seven years before Winnicott's death, at a time of great consolidation of his clinical experience. The girl was seen fourteen times over two and a half years, until she was five years old. Throughout this treatment, the most acute symptoms gradually disappeared. Initially, Piggle had concerns that kept her awake at night, in great distress. It all began with the birth of her younger sister when she was one year and nine months old; before that, she had been a calm child, but then she became depressed, becoming annoyed with everything, manifesting intense anguish and jealousy towards her sister. She told her parents that she now had a black father and a black mother, and she felt that her mother chased her at night and sometimes put her in the toilet.

A second element of Piggle's phantasy referred to an entity that no one could decipher, which she named "babacar". Every night, Piggle begged in despair: "Tell me about the babacar, all about the babacar" (Winnicott, 1977, p. 7). Lost, the only inference the parents could make was that often, the black mother and the black father appeared together, associated with the baba-car, and as a result, Piggle also turned black, ceasing to be who she was.

Piggle suffered greatly, had no more concentration in her play, and hardly admitted to being herself. She then began to ask not to be called Piggle anymore, as she had disappeared, gone away, to the babacar. "Piga is black. Both Pigas are bad." (Winnicott, 1977, p. 7). Her parents no longer knew how to help her. They then told their daughter that they had written to a person, Dr. Winnicott, who understood about "babacars and black mummys", and the girl asked: "Mummy take me to Dr. Winnicott" (Winnicott, 1977, p. 7).

In the first consultation, there was an initial interaction with Winnicott, and some conversations and play about the little sister, the other baby. Then, the mother talked with Winnicott, while Piggle and the father remained in the waiting room. The mother then told Winnicott that Piggle no longer wanted to be herself, preferring to be the mother or the baby. After this first consult-ation, for the first time since the birth of the sister, the parents sent news that Piggle allowed herself to be a baby, entering the "Moses basket" and drinking a huge amount of bottles. She did not admit that anyone else called her Piggle anymore and claimed that the Piggles were bad and black. The girl lay on the bed, crying without knowing why, and told her parents that Dr. Winnicott knew nothing about "babacars". But she said that her teddy-bear did want to go back to London to play with Winnicott, and she didn't, revealing all her ambivalence.

On one hand, Winnicott had helped a lot by allowing Piggle to take on the role of the baby after that session, but he had not been able to decipher the strangeness of the "babacar". The mother was unaware of the exact origin of this term, knowing only that it was associated with the color black, the black self, and black people. In the midst of cheerful events, Piggle suddenly looked worried and said, "The babacar has arrived". This spoiled everything; everything turned black. Nevertheless, after the first session with Winnicott, the parents reported that a good mother started to emerge. However, when she couldn't sleep, it was always because of the "babacar".

In the second consultation, Winnicott asked Piggle twice to explain what the "babacar" was, but she was unable to answer. So, he ventured an inter-pretation: "It's the mother's inside where the baby is born from" (Winnicott, 1977, p. 24) – this is precisely the point we emphasize, which was only possible due to the Kleinian tradition of thought. Piggle looked at Winnicott, relieved, and agreed: "Yes, the black inside" (Winnicott, 1977, p. 24). This interpretation increased the girl's confidence, and the two engaged in a dra-matic play, in which Winnicott had to take on the role of a very voracious baby and Piggle that of the mother of this baby. She began to direct the dra-matic scene, and the analysis began to flow.

The Kleinian intuition that the maternal body is the first geography for a child was present, leading Winnicott to interpret Piggle's unconscious phan-tasy. Indeed, Klein helped us unravel the mysterious and strange nature of the inside of the body, from which babies, milk, words sprout: sometimes lumi-nous, at other times indeed a dark and threatening place, harboring the most unexpected eruptions of pleasure and displeasure, taking us out of our com-fort zone, inventing another baby that comes to share with us the maternal gift that was supposed to be ours alone, exclusively. Therefore, in the first session, Piggle repeated several times the other baby, the other toy, emphasizing the other, the unassimilable event of this arrival, this alterity.

It was Klein's enlightenment desire, her desire to shed light on the darkest corners of human affectivity that made therapeutic efficacy possible in a case like Piggle's, and many others that came after, and those that are still to come.

Notes

1 Our translation.
2 For further exploration: Enactments e transformações no campo analisante (Tamburrino, G., 2016).

References

Baranger, M., & Baranger, W. (2008). The analytic situation as a dynamic field. *International Journal of Psychoanalysis, 89*(4), 795–826. (Original work published in 1961–1962).

Klein, M. (1923). Infant analysis. In: *Contributions to psycho-analysis 1921-1945*. Great Britain: The Hogartth Press Ltd.

Ogden, T. H. (2009). *Rediscovering psychoanalysis – Thinking and dreaming, learning and forgetting*. Routledge.

Ogden, T. H. (2004). *This art of psychoanalysis – Dreaming undreamed dreams and interrupted cries*. Routledge.

Ogden, T. H. (1994). *Subjects of analysis*. Jason Aronson Inc.

Tamburrino, G. (2016). Enactments e transformações no campo analisante. São Paulo: Escuta. (translation: Enactments and transformations in the analytic field).

Winnicott, D. W. (1977). *The Piggle – The Piggle: An account of the psycho-analytic treatment of a little girl* (I. Ramzy, Ed.). Hogarth.

1 A brief overview of Melanie Klein's work

Coming to terms with the soul's wounds

Elisa Maria de Ulhôa Cintra

If I were asked today which psychoanalytic author has contributed the most to our understanding of the deepest and most primitive unconscious functioning, I would have no doubts in answering: Melanie Klein. She teaches us to set aside common sense and restraint to understand the autonomous and demonic nature of unconscious phantasies, whose strangeness challenges us, erupting against our will, possessing us, and seeking expression through us and beyond our control.

The author's clinical cases help to grasp the autonomous nature, the otherness of unconscious functioning in relation to everyday experiences. There is a song by Chico Buarque (1976), "What will be (In full bloom)"[1], which speaks about what "has no measure and never will" – our omnipotent and immeasurable passions, love, jealousy, control, possession, ambition, envy, anger, with their untamed, unlimited, and insatiable character: "which has no governance, and never will". It is a world of desires that overflow, shoot, and threaten to overwhelm us. Faced with the autonomy of unconscious "desires", coming from elsewhere and marginalizing us in relation to our more well-behaved "self", the poet asks himself: "What is it that gives me?" showing his astonishment at the desire that seeks to encompass everything: the fullness of satisfaction, omnipresence, and exclusive possession of the object of love. A grandiose demand for absolute, urgent, unrealizable love, destined for frustration: this is what Klein considers the "infantile" – that is, insatiable – character of all human desiring in its most unconscious and archaic source – the birthplace of anxiety, the most primitive and difficult anxieties to traverse.

The infantile is a dimension outside of time, a threatening backdrop, given the immensity of its demand. A primitive language that has not yet learned to speak (infans means "the one who does not speak") makes an appeal for access to figuration, it wants to be formulated at all costs, it wants to reveal itself. It exists in the most unconscious recess, secret, pulsating, in all psychic processes and at all ages, not just at the beginning of life. Invasive, as it seeks an interpreter who can give it a name and figure: "What is it that gives me?"

DOI: 10.4324/9781003583035-2

Let's listen to the author's voice:

My work has taught me that the first object to be envied is the feeding breast, for the infant feels that it possesses everything he desires and that it has an unlimited flow of milk, and love which the breast keeps for its own gratification: thus it is [also] the first object to be envied by the child. This feeling adds to his sense of grievance [by not receiving what it needs and what it is entitled to] and hate [by the object that refuses to give what it has], and the result is a disturbed relation to the mother. (…) I would not assume that the breast is to him [the baby] merely a physical object. The whole of his instinctual desires and his unconscious phantasies imbue the breast with qualities going far beyond the actual nourishment it affords. We find in the analysis of our patients that the breast in its good aspect is the prototype of maternal goodness, inexhaustible patience and generosity, as well as of creativeness. It is these phantasies and instinctual needs that so enrich the primal object that it remains the foundation for hope, trust, and belief in goodness. (…). But it is equally, as we have seen above, the object that possesses and does not give, generating much envy. This [primary envy] should be differentiated from its later forms (inherent in the girl's desire to take her mother's place and in the boy's feminine position) in which envy is no longer focused on the breast but on the mother receiving the father's penis, having babies inside her, giving birth to them, and being able to feed them.

(Klein, 1957, p. 180–183)

Primary envy

It may seem very strange to speak of the feeling of envy in a newborn, even though it concerns envy of the breast and the physical and psychic sources of nourishment, present from the beginning of life. Freud already defined primary love as the feeling directed towards sources of gratification and nourishment.

The objection raised against Melanie Klein regarding the precocity of envy has often been revisited and discussed. We may admit that the envy consciously felt by an adult is different from this first form, present from the cradle. But it is worth insisting: this infantile envy that operates on an unconscious level and does not come to be "felt" is not the privilege of the baby alone. To a greater or lesser extent, it is within all of us and at times may even dominate our minds.

The primary envy referred to by our author is, in fact, another way of talking about the brute force of desire at its origins. In this sense, to envy is to desire very, very strongly, to the point of wanting to possess what one desires. In French, the word for envy, "envie", also means the desire to have, to possess, to do something in the same way as someone we admire. The desire to possess the loved object can reach the point where the envious one wants to merge with it.

Envy is therefore a primary form, a state of passionate exaltation: the desire to "be the loved person", to merge with them, while feeling, at the same time, the tragic impossibility of interpenetrating them, "being them" from within. Who does not remember the vehement passion of the heroine of Emily Brontë's novel *Wuthering Heights* (1847), declaring, with regard to the beloved man: "I am Heathcliff"! Incorporation and possession phantasy, love in its origins is so infiltrated with primary envy that it is difficult to identify them separately.

The love of the newborn and the love of the adult woman who feels drawn by a phantasy of incorporation and possession of the beloved man are placed side by side here as if there were no significant differences between their protagonists. This shows that we are referring to desires and anxieties in their unconscious dimension and outside of time, as latent possibilities throughout life that can be relived in adulthood. They are therefore outside chronological time in a mythical temporality, of origins and the originating, which remains as a living core, capable of vitalizing or obstructing the opening to affective experiences.

Health and illness

Health or pathology arises from an interplay between antagonistic forces and a relationship between the individual and the welcoming or hostile environment over time. For Melanie Klein, two polarities govern psychic life: the life drive, a tendency that leads to greater integration of the psychic apparatus, and the death drive, a tendency toward disintegration and disorganization through destructiveness. The life drive expresses the investment of love: it leads to the movement of placing libido and interest in people and the world. On the other hand, the death drive corresponds to the lethal tendency of narcissism, that is, the erasure and dissolution of the self and the importance and significance of other people; it is the tendency to disregard others, to become indifferent, to numb sensitivity and perception of emotions, to become callous and closed off.

These two polarities close to instinctual or drive life are energies that, in the human case, very early come into contact with the realm of language and meanings, establishing the human sexuality field as territory of both biology and the need for communication: the newborn comes into contact with the conscious and unconscious sexuality of its peers, its parents, and other adults. It enters a true "magnetic field" that gives rise to an endless tumult of stimuli, sensations, excitements, attractions, and repulsions, or to a true "libidinal bath", which includes beliefs, values, and moral judgments.

Obviously, much of the forces and dynamics that bathe the newborn are enigmatic, strange, intense, and disproportionate to the neonate's capacity for containment or understanding, creating the most foreign aspects of its unconscious. The strangeness of this "vile bargain", which are unconscious phantasies, continues to challenge us throughout life. Such phantasies are, in the realm of unconscious psychic life, the correlates of the affective impulses directed towards their objects of love (life drive) and hatred (death drive).

As we have seen, primary envy, as an unconscious phantasy, is therefore an example of the combination between the life and death drives, the dark and immeasurable side of the vampiric libidinal desire – life drive – or attraction and covetousness, which combine with destructiveness – death drive. The death drive is in the tendency to appropriate the qualities of the other, to diminish their importance, to suppress them; that is, it is a radical form of absolute narcissism that aims to dissolve all differences between the individual and their objects, in order to give the subject the illusion of omnipotence and total independence. With this, they hope to suffer less, to feel less the absence of someone, which, in reality, they cannot achieve with this primitive defense strategy against psychic pains.

Degrading the value of other people, despising them, reveals the fear of suffering and, as it is known, "that's just sour grapes…".

The target towards which envy is directed is the good, the beautiful, the admirable gift of an artist, for example. Envy desires the imaginary possession of creativity, the talent that another person has for generating, that which is most secret and unique in each individual. Envy gives clear expression to the voracity, the greed of desire. The baby approaches the breast like a vampire – it wants to suck everything, and this voracity turns into a desire to strangle and squeeze, to discover everything that is warm and precious in the maternal body, to withdraw all its precious contents and appropriate them. They have a magical character, and the maternal body becomes the concrete and metaphorical horizon of all that is good. Vampiric sexuality realizes the combination of love and the desire to bite the loved object, to tear it into pieces, to cover it with urine and feces, to attack it with poisonous and magical substances, to open this body to see what is inside, to appropriate what is valuable there. Ultimately, it is the excessive ambition of this love that makes it sadistic.

The excessiveness of primitive love

Here is the Kleinian phantasmagoria that led Lacan to call Klein a "brilliant meat butcher", capable of giving name and figure to the most unconfessed sexual and aggressive phantasies. She is an author who invites us to set aside our aesthetic prejudices and the need for a beautiful theory to do precisely this with her: a movement of demotion, of degradation from the abstract to the material and bodily plane, in accordance with Bakhtin's words (1984, p. 19) describing the grotesque style in Renaissance literature:

> To degrade consists in bringing closer to the earth, entering into commu-
> nion with the earth conceived as a principle of absorption and, at the

same time, of birth (...) it means entering into communion with the life of the lower part of the body, that of the belly and genital organs, and therefore with acts such as coitus, conception, pregnancy, childbirth, the absorption of food, and the satisfaction of natural needs. It rushes not only downwards, towards nothingness, absolute destruction, but also towards the productive low, where conception and rebirth take place, and where everything grows profusely.[2]

The Kleinian theory thus approaches the art of the grotesque in this excessive and unabashed advance towards the lowest and darkest regions of the mind, but which are also the most vital and fertile.

Such excess of our most primitive way of loving often remains unconscious, repressed, and unrecognizable by us in our daily lives. It is most common for us to defend ourselves against this "reality" with great horror: "I never felt anything like that". "What an exaggeration!". "How does she know the baby has this?". We can say that, from her analytic sessions with her first child patients and also through adult patients, Klein infers the presence of a sadistic force in the love of origins, with all its share of instinctual violence.

Melanie Klein emphasized Freud's discovery that infantile sexuality – polymorphous and with traces of violence and sadism – is a heterogeneous formation, a "vile bargain" – the nursery of all archaic anxieties (or anguishes).

In a trilogy about the "Female Genius"[3], Julia Kristeva recognizes the importance of Melanie Klein, Hannah Arendt, and Colette – who dared to think, desire, and make their own judgments in a century of barbarism and prejudice. Kristeva (2002) asserts that: "By understanding more clearly than anyone else the anguish, a wave carrying pleasure, Melanie Klein made psychoanalysis an art of caring for the capacity to think."

Transformation of archaic anxieties

We highlight here an important fact: archaic anxieties only transform through a process of thought, called symbolization. This process coincides with psychoanalytic work, which is simultaneously the art of caring, healing, and creating a capacity to think, emancipated from parental figures and mentors. In current times, the independence of thought is under threat; people do not allow themselves to heed the Enlightenment invitation to dare to think for themselves, freeing themselves from a constraining sense of intellectual minority, and unable to take a necessary distance from tradition that would allow them to nourish themselves while simultaneously detaching enough to create something new.

Daring to think for oneself requires a certain fruitful irreverence, a capacity to separate oneself from idols, parents, and mentors. It is precisely what Melanie Klein, as a free and independent disciple of Freud, accomplished in her theoretical work, and it is this same goal that is aimed for in a Kleinian analysis.

Archaic anxieties and the paranoid-schizoid and depressive positions

Let's take a closer look now at what is at stake in Melanie Klein's theorization regarding archaic anxiety situations. In the case of persecutory anxieties, which characterize the paranoid-schizoid position, anxiety is considered archaic due to its tone of persecution, fear of being attacked and invaded as revenge for all phantasies of appropriating the maternal body, in the passionate fury of cruel love. The law of retaliation – an eye for an eye, a tooth for a tooth – will be responsible for the return upon oneself of the sadistic desires of primitive love.

Clinical observations regarding the earliest stages of life led Klein to emphasize the mode of relation in pre-genital stages, a moment when there is still no capacity to care for and be concerned about the other person, who is not even recognized in their autonomous and separate existence. "Unable to recognize the rights, needs, or desires of the object, it ends up being merely something to be consumed and therefore destroyed, or something to be controlled and subjugated. In this case, the 'law of the jungle' prevails, the one that orders 'grab, kill, and eat'" (Cintra and Figueiredo, 2004, pp. 62–63).

What is at stake at this moment is, therefore, the very life of the desiring subject, voracious, envious, and destructive. Therefore, such anxieties are called annihilating anxieties.

> In opposition to this "law of the jungle", a "law of culture and society" may later be established, a moment of recognition of the object as another desiring subject, in which libidinal drives will prevail, and a capacity to recognize the other as autonomous and as a center of subjectivity with their own needs and desires may develop. (...) Between six and nine months of life, when the child has become capable of recognizing the mother, the mere appearance of a stranger in her place is enough to trigger that anxiety that we relate to the danger of loss of the object.
>
> (Cintra and Figueiredo, 2004, p. 68)

Such anxieties of loss will be called depressive anxieties, for here the subject fears having spoiled or even destroyed, with their sadism and their pulsional urgency, the best things in the world: their good objects.

Thus, recognizing the other person as someone alike and at the same time autonomous, with the possibility of absence and return, is the other major source of archaic anxieties recognized by Freud and Melanie Klein. Such anxiety is difficult to bear when the individual blames themselves for the absences, damages, or death of lost objects. The possibility of the other person disappearing, of ceasing to be interested and solicitous, and ultimately of dying is unbearable, becoming then a source of depressive anxiety.

Since the Three Essays on the Theory of Sexuality (1905) and throughout his work, Freud spoke of a situation that is experienced repeatedly, from the moment the infant begins to recognize the difference between their mother and other adults. If the child finds themselves in a state of helplessness and in need of something they cannot obtain on their own, from nourishment to a little comfort and affection, and there is no one to speak to them, dispelling the darkness of the room, then maternal absence turns into a feeling of being abandoned. The anxiety about loss is confirmed, while the demand for love continues to pulse and demand satisfaction: this creates an atmosphere of insecurity, sadness, and terrible suspicions of being responsible for the aban-donment, an invisible cause of misfortune. It is the terrible fear of being one of those responsible for the ruin of good things, for possessing within oneself something spoiled or death-generating.

Depressive anxiety – a mixture of longing, grief, pain, shame, anger, and the sense of having harmed and been harmed – is the most difficult suffering to bear because it combines guilt, a feeling of self-depreciation for not having prevented the catastrophe, and a sense of powerlessness to avoid evil and loss; this is the archaic anxiety of the depressive position.

One of the greatest psychic torments and one of the most difficult tasks of this subjective position is to accept the vulnerable, dependent human con-dition subject to deception, flaws, illusions, and all kinds of frustrations and hopes. On the other hand, losses, when accepted and processed, lead to growth, maturation, broadening of perspectives, and expanding the possi-bility of using what nature has given us.

Mourning, elaborating the loss

But what does it really mean to mourn or to perform the symbolic work of processing loss? A first answer is: to acquire the ability to process or digest the excess of emotions linked to loss and to engage in temporal processes, humanizing oneself. Let's start with the example of a child who loses their father and feels completely devastated and resentful. The anxiety, guilt, and suffering combined with anger, powerlessness, and feelings of humiliation and helplessness make it very difficult to accept, digest, and modify the emotions that have been mobilized.

The wound of loss needs to be healed, the wound needs to be "thought". Doctors use remedies and bandage. The analyst, a doctor of emotional wounds, can help in another way – by accompanying the person, listening to them, dedicating time to them, inviting them to take a certain distance from events in their factual brutality, and developing with them words and thoughts about themselves and the world that act as "soul remedies", so that they can transform some emotions.

Although the transformed emotions remain what they are: love, hate, envy, shame, guilt, etc., they become digestible and add color and richness to psy-chic life. This is because the pain changes when the wounded person begins to be listened to attentively and can report the repercussions of the events on their psyche, developing a dialogue that allows for a change in understanding of the events. Something seems to deepen or gain nuances. A new perspective is built, and within the new framework, some things expand, others reduce; there is a rearrangement of positions, and an insight emerges. Insight is a new view of the facts, constructed uniquely by the wounded person. This pain, when thought about, is a place of new creation. This creation, in turn, helps to take the treatment a little further. After all, to create is also to repair real or imaginary damage; to create is also to be able to thank for what one has received: "when life gives you lemons, make lemonade".

The entire Kleinian analysis aims to expand the individual's capacity to creatively repair and be grateful. In the end, repair and gratitude are the great healers of the diseases of the soul.

Healing psychic pains, as mentioned above, is not about numbing one-self. On the contrary, it is about expanding the capacity to endure them and transforming them for one's own benefit and for the benefit of others. The Kleinian treatment of primitive anxieties has an undeniable ethical dimen-sion. When this becomes possible, contact with pain, instead of mutilating or neurotically blaming, makes the wounded person more capable of taking an active stance; they feel compelled to discover their own way to "bounce back". Being active, transforming pain into something interesting, eliminates the fear of being passive; it opens up the possibility of feeling more vividly and sharply and of surrendering to this new experience – that of being a sen-sitive sounding board for the emergence of psychic life in all its shades.

Gradually, it is possible to lose the shame of feeling psychic pain, because it only diminishes and inspires after being embraced, lived, and "thought about". The pains and losses are not properly resolved, but they can be traversed in more creative and intelligent ways. The pain of loss then ceases to be experienced as punishment and becomes an opportunity to be more alive, in a much more vibrant contact with the physical and social world. It is a slow journey, teaching one to enter into temporal processes and to know duration, waiting. Many "pennies" only drop later, when there is time to make the connection between what has been experienced and a world of memories, words, stimuli, and past and present sensations. It is necessary to dream loss, death, and situations of loneliness. The stark reality of death is very brutal, leading to nothing. It needs to be brought into a field of meaning to become acceptable. Raw, archaic anxiety is an overwhelming amount of affect without face and name; monstrous. By dreaming it, it connects with words, play, becoming secondary anxiety, softer and more bearable.

So, we learn to wait and see how things will turn out, despair diminishes, and a kind of weak hope emerges, still accompanied by a sense of helpless-ness. The feeling of being fragile, vulnerable does not go away, forcing us to find a way to give positive value to human fragility, associating it with some gain, making us more sensitive and humane. All of this is what we commonly call "going through mourning"; it is losing to gain delicacy, insight, new ways of feeling pleasure, and making contacts.

It seems elementary, but we hardly manage to go through all of this alone; the process requires the company of someone who can support the journey without interfering too much, without becoming too anxious and hurried. Mourning is a common procedure, similar to biological digestion; it exists to "let the past go" and to open up the future. However, despite being so basic, it mobilizes such an unbearable amount of affects that it is something we try to escape through every possible and imaginable means.

However, by avoiding it, we lose contact with the world and plunge into depression, manic-depressive states, and melancholy.

Thus, those who do not feel the pain and do not mourn their infantile and megalomaniacal omnipotent expectations fall into depression, in the pathological sense. Often, this melancholic depression is confused with a good and healthy capacity for sadness: one must be able to feel sad about what is being lost, what is left behind, but without which life stagnates and repeats, without anything new emerging ahead. The "depressive position", when properly traversed, leads to the ability to feel sad without despairing.

Is the process of elaborating the depressive position endless?

This is the Kleinian paradox: the depressive position exists to be traversed and overcome, not once, but thousands of times, because human life demands that it be remade as many times as there are losses. When traversed in the manner described above, it becomes the best antidote to depression, creating antibodies that protect us from melancholic and depressive tendencies.

Losses occur all the time from the moment we are born, including all the changes in state demanded by growth, such as losing the intrauterine situation and having to undergo changes in metabolism, habits, and way of life. Losing the "comfort" of early childhood, the cuddles, the bottle, the attention, the pampering, the diapers, the constant presence of adults around younger children. Entering and leaving schools, changing houses, cities, parents' separation, loss of friends. Children leave behind their most beloved toys, books, clothes, get sick, recover, change bodies, voices. But all these losses are also new opportunities, and Kleinian analysis is aimed at freeing us from a form of pain that blocks access to new opportunities in life.

In listening, Melanie Klein developed the task of discovering how each person positions themselves in the face of their pains, how they deal with their anxiety. What phantasies does this person construct? Do they help or hinder in their arduous, but also so rich and extraordinary, task of continuing to live? Our author observed, then, the "theories" that each person constructs about their situation in the world, a field always open to subtle changes. What threatens the most? Is it the danger of losing someone? Is it the pain of having lost – loved ones, power, prestige, and social status – and feeling implicated in it? Is it, even worse, the despair of seeing their inner and outer worlds threatened with destruction, shattered? Where does the most acute threat fall: the fear of not being sufficiently beautiful, intelligent, healthy? Of being abandoned by everyone, of being humiliated? Is it the bitter impression of having sabotaged oneself, of not being able to fully authorize the use of one's abilities? Is it the resentment of not being helped, of being treated unfairly? All these anxieties at very intense levels disturb and block psychic processes. But it is also they who, when "healed" and transformed, give meaning to our existence.

To map out the internal, unique geography of each person's world, Melanie Klein learned and taught us to listen to the endless narrations and theories that patients weave about themselves and the world, at every moment of their lives and throughout an analysis. Imaginary scripts – night dreams, unconscious phantasies, and daydreams – that make every person a tireless theorizer of themselves and their experiences. How does this singular person position themselves in the face of the fundamental events of their history? How do they undertake the construction of the fabric of phantasies and theories that give meaning to, or destroy, or at least paralyze the meaning of their life? We can see that this restlessness gave rise to the theory of the paranoid-schizoid and depressive positions as presented above.

Finally, if we turn our gaze to Kleinian thought, perhaps the first thing that strikes us in her clinical work is her way of staying close to the experience of suffering and anxiety of the patients. With anxiety, we reach the most basic ground of psychic functioning, we touch what is most visceral, most intimate, most deeply determinant of all psychic organization. Melanie Klein believed this to be the most "neuralgic" thread of analytic listening, the one that leads to the infrastructure of psychic occurrence. The hypothesis is that by listening and intervening in the register of anxiety, we reach the level of the forces that generate psychotic suffering and produce neurosis, in its unconscious and inaccessible dimension.

We can assert, without hesitation, indeed, that without empathetic resonance with the patient's suffering, it is not possible to conduct an analysis or any other relationship.

As we have already pointed out, Klein stands in the lineage of Ferenczi regarding a certain type of listening: firstly, directing attention to the forces that produce conflict and pain, and only in a second moment, discerning the path of deconstructing defenses, ways of being in the world that are preventing, mutilating, and inhibiting the free manifestation of psychic life.

In summary, this is the immense importance of this psychoanalyst for all post-Freudian psychoanalysis, even when not all of her theses and technical procedures are adopted integrally.

Notes

1 NT: A free translation of "O que será (À flor da pele)".
2 NT: translator's rendition.
3 NT: Female Genius is a free translation from the Portugues version entitled "*Gênio Feminino: Melanie Klein*".

References

Bakhtin, M. (1984). *Rabelais and his world*. (H. Iswolsky, Trans). Indiana University Press.

Bronte, E. (1847). *Wuthering heights*. Penguin Books, 2002.

Cintra, E. M. U. and e Figueiredo L. C. (2004). *Melanie Klein: Estilo e pensamento* [Free translation: Melanie Klein: Style and Thought]. Escuta.

Freud, S. (1905). Three Essays on the Theory of Sexuality. In *The standard edition of the complete psychological works of Sigmund Freud, Volume VII (1901-1905): A case of hysteria, three essays on sexuality and other works*. (J. Strachey, Trans.) (pp. 123–246). Imago Publishing.

Klein, M. (1957). Envy and Gratitude. In *Envy and gratitude and other works 1946– 1963*. Free Press, 1984.

Kristeva, J. (2002). *The female genius* (Vols. 1–3). Columbia University Press.

Song reference

Buarque, C. (1976). O que será? (À Flor da Pele) [What could it be? (On edge)] [Song]. In Meus caros amigos [My dear friends]. Philips, Universal Music.

2[1] The Kleinian enlightenment project

Making the invisible visible[2]

Elisa Maria de Ulhôa Cintra

The last hundred years of psychoanalysis have taught us to see psychic functioning through topics, maps and models, initially those created by Freud, Klein, Winnicott, Bion, and others. Their seminal works gave rise to countless more, in a process of multiplication, an interminable flow of invention bent on making the invisible visible. These psychoanalytic models can be transformed into animated film-scripts, and that makes learning theory much more fun!

There would seem to be a real need for discernment, a clearer idea of what is going on inside us in terms of our emotions, memories, and sensations, so that we can live better, stave off all those somber notions, nostalgia for the past and fear for the future, the emotion-overload that invades the body and steals our voice. Reflecting on and symbolizing lived experience is our most intimate "compulsion", and it is also the principle underlying all types of therapy and analysis, the therapeutic action that leads to *insight and healing*. It corresponds to the need to reinvent oneself every single day and to constantly step outside one's comfort zone. Pontalis once said in an interview that to heal oneself is to change place.

Along these same lines, we might say that psychoanalysis has to be invented anew every time, made-to-measure for each new patient and analytical encounter (Ogden, 2005). Bion (1967/2014) teaches us that we need to receive our patients as if every session were the first; in other words, the analyst can never cling to what he or she already knows but must constantly search for what has not yet come to mind. Every session is unique, and it is interesting how each new encounter yields transformations, even if they are only microtransformations, to use Ferro's term (2005).

To all intents and purposes, our curiosity about what is going on psychically can be traced back to the very start of life: natural born theorists of the self, others and the events of life and death, we create our blueprints of the psychic apparatus.

Thinking of psychic life through unconscious fantasies, the scenarios those fantasies present and the internal objects encountered therein, Melanie Klein was the first analyst to stress so clearly the visual dimension of psychic life,

DOI: 10.4324/9781003583035-3

which could be compared, in a sense, to the stream of images in a film. Another central aspect of her thought, as we have seen, is the idea and process of mourning that comes with the depressive position, and that is why we have opted to speak at length about an animated film that explores the emotional experience of loss and mourning in the life of a young girl named Riley.

This refers to the animation *Inside Out*[3], which takes us to "look inside the mind of an eleven-year-old girl" who had to leave her hometown and move within her own country to a new, strange, and unfamiliar place, stirring up intense emotions, resistance to loss, and grief. The story invites us to observe the workings of the psychic apparatus, which from the outset raises the question: "Have you ever wondered what goes on in someone's mind?"

The animation invites us to exercise imagination and metaphorical capacity – qualities every psychoanalyst needs. In the dark universe of minds, it is necessary to invent models to get a bit closer to this reality, which resists full capture and understanding; theories are always more or less speculative approximations.

Adapting the psychic models of psychoanalysis to suit those of an animated movie may require the over-simplification of models constructed out of careful clinical observation and years of theoretical practice, but we thought it worth a try in this case. When listening to patients as they recount their lives and sufferings, it is essential to allow images to form in association with what is heard. Much in the same manner, it seems to us that *Inside Out* looks to lend "image and form" to the inner world of this eleven-year-old girl as she rides the storm of intense grief and separation.

The construction of the *animation* around a single life episode works well, as it abandons the aim of understanding everything and dives into a main event, which becomes a kind of clinical vignette from which interesting hypotheses and insights can be drawn.

The movie invites us to exercise our imaginations and metaphoric capacity, qualities which every psychoanalyst needs to have. In the dark universe of minds, we must invent models that help us move ever closer to this reality, which does not allow itself to be fully grasped or known; theories can only ever be speculative approximations, and even then with varying degrees of success.

One hundred and fifteen years of psychoanalysis have gone by since the publication of *The Interpretation of Dreams*. Freud (1900/2024) was one of the first to dream, to lend name and form to *psychic reality*. He helped us to see that psychic life is real, despite our denials; in fact, it is every bit as actual as material reality. Invisible though it may be, its effects are concrete and palpable, and become matter and memory, life and death, comfort and attack. Moreover, the psychic is what emotion stirs and memory registers: the root of suffering, for example, can often be imaginary only, but its effect is very real indeed. The pain is actual pain, and we feel it throughout the body, head to toe. It pervades us, and makes us scream and cry, beseech and implore. Conversely, it can shock us into silence, as pain generates a defense mechanism that erases everything, until we find ourselves sedated, as if by general anesthetic.

To picture and represent *psychic reality*, Freud invented two topics, two theories of drive, two theories of angst, describing dozens of defenses and mechanisms through which emotions either boil over or are contained, become available to thought or are mortally erased, lost to all representation.

Since Freud, Melanie Klein has shown that we create characters and the-atrical settings in fantasy: these internal objects can animate us and make us live, or they can deflate, stifle, and crush us until we lose the will to go on. With Winnicott we learned to see the subjective objects that make up our most archaic and hallucinatory psychic reality, breaking out of our dark inner world into outer life, and finding tangible, huggable form in dolls, teddy-bears, and comfort blankets.

Part of these analysts' work has always been the effort to *see*, to lend visi-bility to the invisible. Their job is to produce theories, semantic in origin, that bring the unseeable into sight, because sight enhances hearing and understanding. Hence the fact that some analysts listen as if filming what they are being told.

Back to the film, *Inside Out* begins with a question posed by a girl's voice, asking if one has ever observed someone and wondered what might be happening inside their mind. The same voice then responds confidently, expressing that she knows the answer. This is the inner voice of eleven-year-old Riley, the main character, an I-narrator who weaves the imaginary stories of life; the "character" in each of us that confers consistency on this volatile existence. What consistency? How illusory is that! So much is ignored that can never become voice and word, but remains gagged in the unconscious, and, in our day-to-day lives, mired in the darkness of unsayable sensations and corporeal memories. Yes, that is true...But it does not stop that *raw psy-chic material* from making its demands, fighting its way out of silence in order to form this voice; a voice through which to build a narrative arc, cobble together past, present, and future, weave emotions and reach for the words to express sensations.

In the film, Riley's voice narrates how things came to pass right from the dawn of consciousness. When Riley was born, her psyche was a small, dark, largely unfurnished and uninhabited room. In the center of this space stood a command center consisting of a single button, which, when pressed, triggered the onset of psychic life; a life built out of experiences and mem-ories. But who is responsible for this inaugural moment? We hear the voice of the I-narrator, who takes shape as the character Joy. We might go with Freud and associate this internal character with *libidinal vitality*, surging from our very first experiences of pleasure. At the start of life, we hurtle between extremes of pleasure and displeasure: the inner life of a newborn is this rela-tively unorganized set of intense, either-or fluctuations. Psychic life, properly speaking, is yet to emerge[4].

Joy recounts how the girl's first pleasant memory was created, eleven years before. She'd opened her eyes to find herself held in the loving gaze of her besotted parents. Their beaming smiles, the sound of their voices and words served as a sort of mirror full of echoes and reverberations in which she saw herself for the very first time. Looking at her, they reflect her back at herself. It's in that instant that psychic life begins.

We see a ray of light shine into the dark room of the psyche. It is life's first narcissism, generating and releasing the power of Eros. Riley embarks on the unending adventure of being seen and recognized. When she looks at her parents, she perceives her own reflection in them and experiences a sense of existence through their gaze. The shiny reflective surface of their doting eyes wields a tremendous power of attraction, drawing her into them, to meld with them. Thus begins the symbiosis of love which will leave unforgettable marks. The desire to be recognized will never fade; it might be partially appeased, but there will always be the indelible mark of lack, and the memory of a happy ghost that passed away leaving her wanting more. The narcissism that is born out of this will forever carry a denial of the rupture and of the passage of time; it is, itself, infinite narcissistic time. From this point on, this first rapture will be sought in each new romantic passion, every trip or vacation, in every feeling of wonderment before natural beauty, or a work of art, or a marvel of science or thought.

During the first five years of life, the whole experience of intimate bodily connection with the mother can be termed primary maternal experience. The most tragic event in life is when this does not occur. Yet even when it happens satisfactorily, it always leaves a sense of nostalgia, as we always want more. Some basic failure persists and will leave a lack – the most painful narcissistic wound – generating an eternal longing for what did not happen, or what did not happen sufficiently.

The loving mirror needs to devolve Riley's own image, give her the sense that she truly exists and help her diminish the feeling of estrangement that comes with thrownness into this existence, the condition of *being-there*, of being inexplicably hurled into the extraordinary experience of finding oneself alive, without forewarning or instruction manual. Having her image reflected back at her is the jubilation of feeling whole and recognized.

In the film, Joy is the first emotion present at the dawn of psychic life. Others will come. In psychoanalytical terms, we might see her as an experience of life instinct, the desire for pleasure, for that which set our psychic life in motion, becoming thereafter the first principle of every investment we make in the world and in others. In a sense, Joy was already there, in that dark space that preceded psychic life. She was there as pure potentiality, but only came into being when woken by the gaze and words of Riley's parents, summoning her out of the darkness. Might Joy perhaps be the life instinct steered by a yet incipient I, an Ibody? Joy is the source of the potential to love and invest in the world, in sexuality, and the capacity to create psychic life. As we shall see further on, the editing table that appears in the film as an emotion-processing desk is, in a sense, the ego and its organizing function.

In response to the loving gaze, Joy presses the only button in the psychic command room and creates the first pleasurable memory, which leaves a trace and sets the psychic mechanism in motion. Psychic life is a great work that begins this way, with furrows and mnemonic traces. The first memory trace opens a passage or facilitation; events carve paths in memory, as if forming riverbeds through which libido flows. The greater the circulation, the deeper the furrow, and the more abundant the river of libido that flows through it, forming associations, intersections, trails, and eventually landscapes imbued with pleasure or pain.

In the movie, a yellow sphere, representing Riley's first core memory, a luminous and joyous glass ball blown by her parents' doting gaze and Riley's response to it, rolls into scene along a conveyor rail. It's fun to think of our circuit of drives beginning in this way, like marbles on a track. It is raw psychic material leaving its first marks, instilling the hunger to someday become word, figure, and narrative. The first mnemic traces are pre-verbal – sensations and feelings – and they inaugurate the demand for symbolization. The lived wants to be spoken one day.

The film depicts the advent of the process of symbolization in the form of a larger editing table that is now controlled by several personified emotions, each given its own color. In the beginning, the table was small, but it has since complexified into a powerful processor of emotions and meanings, operated by Joy, Sadness, Fear, Anger, and Disgust. These are the emotions that will now drive and color Riley's experiences.

The girl's emotional experiences are organized into *sectors* called *inner islands* – the island of family, the island of humor, the island of honesty, the island of friendship, and the island of work and study. These islands are clusters of affects and ideas, relationships with people, and meaningful lived experiences. The family island closely resembles the Oedipal structure described by Freud, a set of ideas intensely invested with affects, desires, expectations, ideals, and identifications. Klein would say that the islands are webs of unconscious phantasies and meanings associated with various aspects of life. These networks of meanings and affects weave and organize psychic life. She speaks of the Oedipus complex as a **situation**, endowing it with the quality of a scene, or multiple scenes that may repeat and transform throughout life and analysis.

Each experience generates memory, and the memories start clustering in associative networks, organized around emotions. In the film, Joy, Sadness, Fear, Anger, and Disgust compete for command over the editing table, and each memory created takes on a color indicative of the core emotion evoked in its production. Yellow is for joy, blue for sadness, purple for fear, red for anger, and green for disgust. As time goes by, memories are stored in mnemic warehouses, where the "Forgetters" inspect the stock and hoover up the more faded memories with a special vacuum cleaner, consigning them to oblivion in the memory dump.

When Riley loses the sense of belonging that connected her to her hometown, she becomes depressed and feels intense anger toward herself and the world: at this moment, the islands that structured her psychic functioning "collapse". In psychoanalytic terms, depression is a psychic collapse; there is a withdrawal of libido, which falls into the abyss of self-depreciation, and in the depressed individual, there is a general movement of disengagement from the world and a profound unconscious anger corresponding to this internal collapse. It is deeply sad to see everything falling apart.

After the fall, the film shows the moment when the girl begins to process her pain and rebuild her internal world on new foundations. Each experience of mourning involves this reconstruction. The fallen islands must be rebuilt, one by one, and they become more complex. A psychic expansion occurs as Riley emerges from her depression, thanks to the working-through of grief and the process of integrating lived experiences that will shape the psychic subject.

During depression, however, as Riley idealized her life up north and detested everything about San Francisco, her expectations fell like a shadow over the ego, revealing an internal world in ruins, with libido flowing straight into an abyss, the "Memory Dump".

Losses, frustrations, and growth

In the first part of the film, seen from inside Riley's psychic apparatus and internal world, we're given a recap of the preceding eleven years of the character's life up north in Minnesota, where most of her memories have been happy and luminous, with joy predominating. Happy family moments, her growing skill on the ice, the pleasure she derives from playing on her ice-hockey team, her play friends, and school life. She has not yet experienced any significant losses or suffering.

When she has to move town and leave her friends and school behind, and the joys of early childhood with them, she embarks on the quest of having to deal with the pain of loss and with mounting frustrations. At this point, Sadness and Joy find themselves overworked, and they end up banging heads a lot. One of these clashes results in the pair being sucked out of the Psychic editing table and deposited in some strange and inhospitable part of the psyche: the unconscious, perhaps? Lost in this uncanny and inhospitable territory, they struggle to find a way back to the Psychic editing table, and set off on an expedition that takes them through the dream-production studios and along other routes dangerously skirting the Memory Dump. At various times during their peregrination, Joy tries to stop Sadness laying her hands on the memory orbs, because her slightest touch would turn them blue. However, something changes at a certain point, and we see that the only way to mourn properly is to go through all the feelings of anger we've been blocking out.

Joy realizes that Sadness doesn't need to be kept forever at bay; in fact, she has an important role to play in resolving certain impasses. The key change occurs when Joy remembers the time Riley lost a hockey championship and her family and friends gathered round her, hugging her and crying with her, and that it was these embraces that had brought them all together and laid the ground for new joys, now colored a mix of yellow and blue. True, the integration of these emotions generates a sadder kind of joy, but one that's deeper and more real because of it. Fused emotions put us in more authentic contact with ourselves and with others.

The film is about the harsh reality of having to go through feelings of loss and absence, with all the quagmires that involves. In fact, that's the saga of every psychic life – we have to accept changes, though our narcissism will fight it, wanting happiness to last forever in an infinite narcissistic time with no long-distance moves, no illnesses, no aging, and no loss of those we love.

Riley has to deal with growing pains, and with the more specific mourning of having to accept a move away from the city where she was born and lived to the age of eleven, a period full of idyllic, happy memories of skating on the ice and spending time with friends she has had to leave behind. Letting the past be past is the hardest thing, an absolute demand made of us from the day we are born!

Many of us fail in this core task, which Melanie Klein called the development of the depressive position. It's touching to see how the film brings out this central insight. Standing at the bridge of the psyche, Joy always considered herself superior to Sadness and did her best to prevent her from taking control or touching any of Riley's memories. That wasn't hard in those charming early years, when Riley had not yet had to face any significant losses. During those times, Joy mostly succeeded in keeping Sadness at a distance, but, despite even her best efforts, the latter occasionally managed to steal a touch and taint some of those happy memories with her intense shade of blue. Even then, though, Joy could usually snatch them back in time to wipe away the smudge and restore the bright yellow glow. In those early years, we can allow children to be just a little manic…

However, excessive happiness in life can, over time, lead to a persistent and unhealthy manic state. The unfettered pursuit of pleasure and joy means a loss of deep contact with the lived and with meaning. Agitation does not combine with deep feeling. Thought tinged with mania is frenzied, and it steamrolls more profound feelings and meanings. In Ancient Greece, the poets used to say that it was all but impossible to understand oneself and others without having suffered.

In the manic state, pleasure-based relationships are too frenetic to be able to yield true satisfaction. Indeed, they can only generate more frustration. However, when experiences are lived, they acquire a touch of sadness, the bittersweet recognition that nothing lasts forever, and that the world will never be a playground. It's a realization that brings about an expansion and deceleration that are vital to mental health. Our breathing deepens, and our gaze reaches farther; it's as though we're watching life from a higher vantage point, where horizons are broader and more distant.

In the film, this discovery comes at two different points. Having been sucked out of the Psychic editing table and dumped into the unconscious, as Joy and Sadness try to make their way back to the editing table, the other emotions find themselves in a deadlock: depression takes hold, no-one sees eye-to-eye on anything, the islands crumble into the abyss, and chaos reigns in the psyche. We're in the depths of melancholia, where we're missing the integration which libido and the process of mourning could bring. Anger takes command and fixes an idea in the girl's mind that she should run away from her family and return to Minnesota to recover the childhood she has lost. Unconscious of the pain that this rupture would cause and of the fruitless nature of the endeavor itself (traveling across the country to her former home), Riley boards the bus and takes her seat. But as the coach heads for the freeway, something extraordinary happens: Sadness and Joy make it back to the Psychic editing table.

Only now, Joy has understood the need to have Sadness by her side, operating the bridge with her, and she tells her to take the lead. Sadness frees herself to act and manages to dislodge the idea-bulb, which Anger has gotten stuck in the console, blocking any true contact Riley might have had with her pain and grief. Sadness pulls the lightbulb from the socket, de-bunging the system, and all that mourning floods through Riley. Gripped by the pain of separation from her parents, she aborts her mission to run away, gets off the bus and returns home to share this pain with her family.

And that is the only formula there is for experiencing loss: we have to recognize it and share it. It's tremendously hard to process pain on our own. Shared, unpacked pain becomes lighter, generates the embrace of relief, and tears. And once freed, Joy can make life flow again, restoring Riley's connectedness to the world, but in a way that is deeply transformed: the manic aspect is gone, and the acceptance and experience of pain was essential in making that happen. In the inner world, after all this work, Sadness and Joy, hand-in-hand, take control of the bridge, and what ensues is considerable psychic growth.

The film shows that, having processed the depressive position, Family, Goofball, Honesty, Friendship, and Hockey Islands have all been rebuilt, bigger and more complex than before. At the same time, a new editing table arrives, with specs for far greater psychic capacity. That's what one should expect of a processed depressive position: more fully integrated emotions; a relinquishing of fixed ideas and omnipotent certainties; the shedding of the absolute ideas of early childhood, a willingness to let the past be the past; and a deeper capacity to feel and think about life.

Earlier on in the film, Joy finally understands the danger of her turning into a manic defense if she keeps on blocking Sadness. This happens when the pair are still lost in the unconscious, during the depressive episode. Far removed from consciousness, Joy meets the long-lost Bing Bong, Riley's old imaginary friend. He's a big pink plush toy, a mix of elephant, cat, and dolphin. Bing Bong is found roaming alone among the racks of stored memories. He laments the pain of having been forgotten by Riley, and receives a comforting embrace from Sadness, much to Joy's surprise. Bing Bong bursts into floods of tears, which are actually sweets and candies that gather around him on the floor. What most catches Joy's attention in this is that, after hugging and having a good cry, Bing Bong and Sadness start smiling again, recomposed on a deeper level. This teaches Joy that sadness is something that can be felt and overcome when shared, just as occurred that time when Riley's pain drew her family and friends around her, fostering a profound communion that resulted in restored joy. There is something sweet in shared tears.

But, despite this realization and all her efforts to return to conscious-ness, there comes a moment that sees Joy slump into an even deeper level of unconsciousness, the Memory Dump, where there is no way back to the upper levels, much less the editing table at the Psychic editing table. She is lost now among the most faded, forgotten memories, in an inhospitable, hopeless netherworld thick with black soot. Together, she and Bing Bong, who has fallen in with her, hatch a plan to fly out of the pit in his old rocket cart, propelled by the familiar tune from their past games that celebrates his playful companionship.

They dig up the half-buried cart, jump in, power it up with some song fuel, and try to fly it back to the upper regions of the psyche, belting the childhood tune out as they go. But their combined weight is too much to get them there, and they succumb to the drag of nostalgia with each attempt. After repeated failures, they are back where they started, at the bottom of the Memory Dump. But on the third or fourth attempt, something magical happens: Bing Bong climbs into the rocket with Joy and helps her gain enough momentum before slipping out half-way up. He decides to sacrifice his own return to con-sciousness so that Joy can succeed, and so allows himself to fall back into the abyss. Lighter without him, the rocket carries Joy back to what is presumably the sub-conscious, or pre-conscious. From there, reunited with Sadness, and with the help of some imaginary childhood boyfriends, Joy is able to catapult herself back to the Psychic editing table, arriving at just the crucial moment, the nadir of the story, when Riley has run away from home and is already on the bus to Minnesota.

It's Riley's childhood imaginary friend and first crushes who provide the energy required to bring her out of depression, but they are all lost in the act. Together, Joy and Bing Bong would have continued to succumb to the gravity of regressive nostalgia and plunged back into the Memory Dump every time. Once the rocket lands on the ledge of the upper regions, Joy calls out to Bing Bong, only to realize he's not with her. She gazes down into the Dump and sees him waving back at her with a slowly disappearing arm. One arm goes, then another, until his whole body vanishes into oblivion, and all so that Joy can return to consciousness with renewed libidinal drive for life. In the

Making-of, we're told that the disclosure of Bing Bong's fate caused quite a consternation among the team.

Looking down from the ledge, Joy sees her friend's body fade away, dissolving into that cold, harsh atmosphere of oblivion. This is the scene that reminds us of what Winnicott called the transitional object of infancy, which helps us through the transitions necessary to the child's development, but which must disappear in order for the maturational process to continue. Joy had to reconnect with her childhood friend, flush with the libidinal energies and oldest experiences of joy and pleasure, in order to get through her impasse. But here, again, there is a lived sadness. As he vanishes, Bing Bong generates just enough energy to send Joy back into consciousness[5].

The work of the psychic apparatus

The film teaches us the essential core of Klein's thought: that the function princeps of the psychic apparatus is to metabolize pain and create pathways and meanings in order to process losses. At the end of the movie, as described above, the islands are rebuilt larger than ever, and some health technicians deliver and install a state-of-the-art editing table that sports a mysterious new button called "puberty". Riley has no idea the world of trouble that's going to cause when pressed, and all the new challenges and losses that lie ahead.

The memories, which were all one color at the start of the film, are now multi-colored, and work on developing the depressive position has progressed significantly. The story reveals that tears when shared can be sweet, and that losses have to be overcome in order to open up new landscapes across which life can continue. Following Gaston Bachelard (1969), we sense here the fundamental role of the other in this process and in mental health as a whole: we move through life in a kind of slumber, enveloped in a world of unconsciousness, until the presence of another reaches us, offering the spark that awakens us into being. It is in this encounter that we are shaped, as before it, we remained undefined, little more than inert existence.

The subject is built through the You – it's a fundamental notion brought to us by Freud, Klein, Bion, Winnicott, and other psychoanalysts. Not only at the moment of its advent, but throughout life, the I is made and remade from the influence of others, who it metabolizes and emulates. In analysis, the subject opens herself up to be built and rebuilt.

The analysand must accept herself in her fundamental condition of dependence and abandonment; accept herself in her state of confusion and paradox, where she is vulnerable and exposed to pain, pleasure, and a host of the most intense passions and angst. That is the human being's true psychic reality. Everything we do to cover that up and deny it is just a defensive strategy. There is a type of excessive joy that transforms into manic defense; and that, in turn, is a mechanism designed to deny sadness. It shows disdain for the human condition in all its vulnerability and finitude, when what we really need is to root ourselves in existence through successive processes of mourning and growth.

These ideas are central to the psychoanalytic process as set forth in such scholarly works as *Mourning and Melancholia* (Freud, 1917/2024) and Klein's writings on mourning (1935, 1940), but they can also be playfully intuited through the animated film *Inside Out*.

Notes

1 This chapter was revised by Eduardo Jefferson de Oliveira, cmo.edu@gmail.com
2 Text presented at the Integration Week of the College of Human and Health Sciences at PUC-SP in November 2015, in a panel coordinated by Ivelise Fortim, with the participation of Professors Denigés, João Perosa, and Luiza Oliveira.
3 *Inside Out* is an animated movie created by Pixar Animation Studios and released by Walt Disney Pictures in 2015. It was directed by Pete Docter and Ronaldo Del Carmen.
4 The book *Virando Gente – a história do nascimento psíquico* (Becoming Human – the Story of Psychic Birth) [2014], written by the psychology professors Ivanise Fontes, Maísa Roxo, Maria Cândida S. Soares and Sara Kislanov, tells the story of a baby starting from inside the womb. (São Paulo: Ideias e Letras).
5 This scene is reminiscent of the part in the German American film *The NeverEnding Story* (1984), directed by Wolfgang Petersen, in which the hero rides his horse into the Swamps of Sadness, where they begin to sink in the mud. Before both can disappear, the horse convinces the hero to continue alone. The horse accepts its fate, but the hero soldiers on, because he has a light in him that prevents him from sinking in the Swamps of Sadness.

References

Bachelard, G. (1969). *The poetics of space*. Boston: Beacon Press.
Bion, W. R. (1967/2014) Notes on memory and desire. In: *The complete works of W. R. Bion*. London: Karnac. Edited by Chris Mawson and editorial consultancy by Francesca Bion.
Ferro, A. (2005). *Fatores de doença, fatores de cura*. Translation: Marta Petricciani. Rio de Janeiro: Imago. (Translation: Factors of illness, factors of healing).
Freud, S. (1900/2024). The interpretation of dreams. In: *The revised standard edition of the complete psychological works of Sigmund Freud*. Translated by James Strachey and revised by Mark Solms. London: Rowman and Littlefield.
Freud, S. (1917/2024). Mourning and melancholia. In: *The revised standard edition of the complete psychological works of Sigmund Freud*. Translated by James Strachey and revised by Mark Solms. London: Rowman and Littlefield.
Klein, M. (1935/1975). A contribution to the psychogenesis of manic-depressive states. In: *Love, guilt and reparation and other works*. New York: Dell Publishing.
Klein, M. (1940/1975). Mourning and its relation to Manic-Depressive States. In: *Love, guilt and reparation and other works*. New York: Dell Publishing.
Ogden, T. H. (2005). *This art of psychoanalysis – Dreaming undreamt dreams and interrupted cries*. London; New York: Routledge.

Pontalis, J-B. (1988/1991) *Perder de vista. Da fantasia de recuperação do objeto perdido*. Translation: Vera Ribeiro. Rio de Janeiro: Jorge Zahar Editor. (translation: Losing Sight: On the Phantasy of Recovering the Lost Object).

Film reference

Inside Out. (2015). Pixar Animation Studios. Directed by Pete Docter; screenplay by Pete Docter, Meg LeFauve and Josh Cooley. Walt Disney Studios Motion Pictures.

3 The genius of child analysis and its implications in clinical practice

Elisa Maria de Ulhôa Cintra and
Marina F. R. Ribeiro

Klein's first and most revolutionary contribution to the contemporary clinic, certainly the one most assimilated by countless psychoanalysts, was the discovery of the analysis of children. This practice, which in the 1920s was seen as daring, soon became a daily reality in the clinic. But how did this happen?

This story begins with Klein's own analytic experience with Sándor Ferenczi in 1914. When Klein was suffering from depressive episodes and had difficulty performing her role as a mother, Ferenczi helped her to look into not only herself but also the psychic universe of her children, incentivising her to analyze her youngest, who suffered from intellectual and affective inhibitions. From this moment, for the first time, the possibility of professional fulfilment became available to the young mother, who had dreamed of becoming a doctor but had found herself incapable of realizing this after marrying and having three children.

In 1918, Klein presented her first psychoanalytic paper, the case study of Fritz (1918–1921), based on observation and analysis of her own son, whose identity was at first anonymous. At the time, the fact of her practice on her own child did not cause a stir since psychoanalysis was still in its inaugural stages. From this first foray into the work of analysis, which opened the doors of the Hungarian Psychoanalytic Society to Klein, she did not stop thinking, writing, and practicing until the end of her life.

The case study of Fritz marks the beginning of the psychoanalytical technique through play. Klein became sensitive to the fact that children express their most profound anxieties and fantasies through play, in which they realize free association. This gave birth to a psychoanalysis of children that excluded all pedagogical elements (Hinshelwood, 1989).

During the session, Klein would actively engage in the fantasy proposed by the child and would speak in the child's own language, always being clear and direct about her hypotheses about the symbolic meaning of play (Hinshelwood, 1989).

The analysis of Rita[1] (1923) was another landmark in the rise of the analysis of small children. Klein began her work with Rita at the family home of the patient, but soon realized it would be more adequate to establish a

DOI: 10.4324/9781003583035-4

different space altogether for the analytic session. Initially, Klein used her own children's toys, and later proposed the use of a designated toy box.

In the words of Klein (1955/1975, p. 129), the analyst:

> (...) should enable the child to experience his emotions and phantasies as they come up. It was always part of my technique not to use educative or moral the influence, but to keep to the psycho-analytic procedure only, which, to put it in a nutshell, consists in understanding the patient's mind and in conveying to him what goes on in it.

The simplicity, relevance, and usefulness of this proposed method are surprising. Beginning with her clinical observations, Klein (1955/1975) understood that a child's inhibition during play represented a serious disturbance, because it reflected a difficulty in forming and using symbols, as well as a perturbance in the world of phantasy. She observed that these children with intellectual inhibitions presented excessive, non-assimilated aggressive impulses, triggering an interest in the clinical and theoretical investigation into the processes of symbolization. How does the capacity to think through what has been experienced come about? For Klein, symbolization has its roots in a primordial interest in one's own body; moreover, the pleasure and pain associated with objects and people in the outside world acquire a proto-symbolic function. The process of figuring and representing lived experience sets in motion the creation of an internal world, of the first wefts of the fabric of unconscious phantasy, a concept we approach in the following chapter.

Indeed, at present, we continue to work with this easy and simple diagnostic criterion: inhibitions in a child's capacity for play indicates psychic suffering and requires care.

Klein's great insight was the realization that play, games, the stories children make up and the comments they make or avoid making can be listened to as one listens to the free associations of adult patients on the couch. Using the child's language to interpret their conflicts and anxieties produces therapeutic effects that can be observed in the emotional and intellectual life of the child and in their social relations.

To conclude this point, and comment on the richness of play, we invoke Manoel de Barros (2010):

A little poem in play-language

He had the dream of a lost bird across his face.
He spoke in bird-language and in child-language.

He was happier playing with words than he was thinking with them.
He passed up on thinking.

When he walked up to the tree he wanted to bloom.
He preferred to make florets out of words than make ideas out of them.

He had learned in the Circus, time ago, that words
must get to toy-level
before they are serious enough to laugh at.

He told his friends that a certain frog had leaped onto one of his
sentences
And the sentence didn't even buckle.
Certainly it did not buckle because there were no bad words in it.

As the boy told the story of the frog over the sentence
In came a Lady by name of Logic von Reason.
The Lady had a walking stick and high heels.
Upon hearing the story of the frog over the sentence the Lady said:
"That's Play Language and it's childish idiocy
For sentences are dreamed-up words, they are weightless, they are not
like ropes, strong enough to hold a frog"

"That's Root-Language" she continued
"It's Make Believe-Language
It's play-language!"

But the boy had the dream of a lost bird across his face
He also wanted to throw some little rocks at common sense.

And he threw rocks:
He said that even today he had seen the Afternoon sit on a tin can
just like a robin sits on a roof tile.

Soon came in Lady Logic von Reason and boomed:
But tin cans cannot handle the Afternoon, and what's more the tin can
has not the space to hold an Afternoon inside it!
That's play-language
It's nothing.

The boy proclaimed:
If Nothingness disappears poetry is done for.
And he crawled into himself like a tortoise.

Developments in analytic method

From the moment the analytic method was opened to children, it became
possible to consider it in relation to cases of psychosis, autism, and borderline. Klein brought forward new clinical proposals, new therapeutic strategies, and a new way of working. Her technique is essentially Freudian: the
interpretation of the unconscious. An unprejudiced attitude toward the primitive aspects of human beings, an attentive mode of listening, an interest in
conflict, in anxieties, in psychic suffering and in the absurdity of human existence – the fact that things happen very differently to how we might like them

to, and that we feel helpless and vulnerable before events, for we can neither predict nor control our own feelings, their intensity, and the reactions of others.

What, then, are the key elements of psychic life that must remain recalcitrant, hidden, outside of consciousness and the possibility of being perceived and elaborated upon? We might think of destructiveness, of sexuality, of singularity and the differences between people; as well as the receptive and feminine capacity to welcome feeling, contemplation, and intuition. Here we might include all desires: envy, hatred, jealousy, the inability to resign oneself to separation, to loss, to the feeling of being slighted or hurt.

Melanie Klein – a kind of radical enlightenment figure, as previously argued – believed in the therapeutic power and curative value of the truth and the possibility of creating an environment that was welcoming and honest, regardless of the age of the patient. Before children, adolescents, and adults alike, the analyst must forsake pedagogical and didactic expectations. Despite her enlightenment approach, the clinical project is not a *civilising* one, but rather one dedicated to deepening and widening one's contact with psychic reality – its impulses, unconscious phantasies, conflicts, pain, and suffering.

Little by little, in an authentically available environment, this contact diminishes the horror patients feel toward psychic life, which in the case of children is the cause of phobias and night terrors. In turn, patients give up their most radical defence mechanisms against their anxieties, mechanisms that are always mutilating. The analyst favors, therefore, finding new ways to make use of and transform both psychic and external realities.

And so, a love of life is not enough; it takes a theoretically informed "intuition" to get in touch with this archaic level of psychic life. This is because, though archaic anxieties might be organized as unconscious phantasies, they have always been outside the field of language, communicating through primitive and pre-verbal means, like projective identification. They consist of the mechanism through which unconscious representations and their affects are projected within the analyst. If the analyst can contain the projected object, they can then help to formulate, in symbolic and linguistic terms, the most archaic anxieties.

The analyst must not imagine that anxieties can be consciously perceived, for they belong to a pre-verbal or pre-narrative layer of the mind. That said, although these anxieties cannot be expressly verbalized, they urgently need to be put to words by *someone*. The analyst must be capable, then, of meeting these archaic anxieties, hold them in their mind and transforming them into a narrative. This is the function of the continence of the mind of the analyst, as Bion called it, such that the analyst can formulate these anxieties into words, opening space for a field of possible symbolizations.

Sometimes, anxieties appear inside out, as a result of defence mechanisms; the patient might say: "I feel nothing", or ridicule the expression of affects, express shame for all that which is related to the body, denoting a repression of sexuality, social phobia, which appears through an excessive reclusiveness and distance, which are schizoid defences. The analyst must name them to access and mobilize the apparition of these buried anxieties and the unconscious phantasies that give them life, and when these anxieties appear, she must go toward them, offering the analytic word – interpretation.

The analyst cannot do this without intuition and empathetic and immediate contact with the world of affects and unconscious representations. She must also be oriented by a theory that explicitly figures the forms in which primitive mental life appears. And so, only when she is able to use a comprehensible narrative language will she be comprehended, even if her analytic ear is tuned to the most abstract and meta-psychological theory. She must, therefore, be attuned to the sonic quality of words, to the semantic and grammatical games that words play, helping the patient to bridge the unrepresentable nature of instinct, the psychic surface and its narratives. She must give name, form, and figure to the unrepresentable instinct, expressed in the unconscious fantasy and which one cannot access through conscious thought. From another point of view, if the analyst remains too convinced of her own theories, of their meta-psychological aspect, she can become intrusive, arbitrary, and violent.

For Klein, the patient needs to do more than to narrate their experiences; they need to re-enact experiences and relational patterns already lived with varying degrees of pleasure at different times in their life and in fact soon begin to help the analyst to do so. What occurs before this enigmatic character, the analyst? Considering that primitive anxieties and their defence mechanisms will be projected onto the analyst, these projections must be left to happen over the course of an analysis, and be worked on through interpretation; but, for this to happen, the atmospheres and the relative positions occupied by the patient and attributed to the analyst by the patient must always be monitored.

Everything the patient does, everything they recount to the analyst, their jokes, their drawings, the dreams they narrate, their comments and associations, their reactions to interpretations offered to them, all appears to be seen and heard as an address to the analyst. The analyst is perceived as a significant figure in the patient's experience and, effectively, put in that position. To a greater or lesser extent, the analyst allows herself to be given this role and, to some degree, incarnates it, really occupying the place the patient puts her in.

Indeed, in the transference, we end up occupying different positions and assuming various roles. No matter who the patient is referring to, we know that, at least in part, it is us they are talking about; it is always us who they address.

The analytical situation is very complex and ends up bringing together many different places, times, and situations, which overlap, unfold, and multiply. The analyst focuses the here and now but is conscious that every "here and now" is a moment of resonance from the past and of anticipation of the future – there is no "here and now" that can be isolated from this overdetermination.

For Kleinians, it is important to recognize that analysis takes place in these conditions and, fundamentally, on these conditions, and it is then a case of interpreting them, discriminating fantasy from reality, past from present, unconscious and conscious. The object of analysis is not the past as it happened, but this complex present, multi-faceted, and overdetermined in which the infant is active, in children and in psychotics, and even in neurotic adults, as a mode of mental functioning, with a form of anxiety, defences, resistances, and ways of relating to internal and external objects.

Analysis is a path that must be traversed so that the patient can be transformed. Often, the analyst is idealized, treated with complacency and too quickly agreed with. Kleinians thus seek to detect the elements of voracity, envy, jealousy, and hatred that are often camouflaged. These destructive elements are inseparable companions to the analytic process, and if they are not interpreted, they will attack everything good and loving that the analyst and the analysis can offer, generating a strong negative therapeutic reaction.

Paying attention to this negative therapeutic reaction – this strange desire not to cure oneself and not to take advantage of what that analysis and that analyst can offer – is something Klein pointed to as decisive, capable of being detected and interpreted from the beginning of the analytic process.

Again, here we see Klein's "radical Enlightenment", according to which these dark forces, opposed to the success of analysis, can be at least in part neutralized, so long as they come to light from the beginning, so that there is not a pact of silence between the patient and the analyst.

Note

1 Although the analysis of Rita occurred in 1923, it was published in 1929 in the chapter titled 'The Psychological Principles of Early Analysis' in Melanie Klein's book *Love, Guilt and Reparation*.

References

Barros, M. (2010). *Poesia completa Manoel de Barros* [Free translation: Complete poetry of Manoel de Barros]. São Paulo: Ed. LeYa.

Hinshelwood, R. D. (1989). *A dictionary of Kleinian thought*. Great Britain: Free Association Books.

Klein, M. (1929/1975). The psychological principles of early analysis. In: Love, guilty and reparation and other works. New York: Delta.

Klein, M. (1955/1975). The psycho-analytic play technique: Its history and significance. In: *Envy and gratitude and other works*. New York: The Free Press.

4 Unconscious phantasy

Contemporary readings

*Elisa Maria de Ulhôa Cintra and
Marina F. R. Ribeiro*

Another of Klein's significant contributions to psychoanalysis is the concept of unconscious phantasy. Though Freud already used the term, it was Klein who deeply investigated the archaic workings of the mind. Indeed, Freud (1923/2024) had postulated that "the ego is first and foremost a bodily ego" (p. 22); however, it was Klein who theoretically and clinically explored the outcomes of the most archaic bodily sensations and their transformation into unconscious phantasy, where the deepest unconscious image of the body is formed.

Sexual instincts, in their various dimensions – oral, anal, urethral – acquire their first psychic representations as unconscious phantasies. For Klein, instincts, as borderline psychosomatic processes, always direct themselves toward objects that can satisfy them. These objects, in turn, transform into "internal objects" of phantasy, forming the internal scenarios that constitute psychic life (Isaacs, 1952/1982; Figueiredo, 2009).

As Cintra and Figueiredo argue (2004, p. 151), "(…) phantasy is the place where one registers what Melanie Klein called 'memories in feelings', but which we could call more precisely memories in *sensations*". It is important, then, that in their daily clinical practice the analyst remains in touch with their own most archaic bodily memories, so that they might capture and resonate with the patient's pre-verbal communications. This is because, if the process of symbolization is interrupted, then unconscious fantasy cannot develop, ties to the external world are impoverished and internal objects are thus concomitantly impoverished. The internal and external worlds become gray, empty, uninhabited.

Klein also contributed to psychoanalytic theory with the conception of an internal world populated by "objects" that might be connected or unconnected to emotion. This was later developed and transformed by Bion into an understanding of "links" (1959/2014).

We might further understand unconscious phantasies as a radical imagination,[1] present in all psychic functions. Phantasy is the process of meaning-making, it is the unconscious psychic life's mode of being and it transforms somatic elements into psychic objects. Phantasy brings instincts, which are

DOI: 10.4324/9781003583035-5

ruled by intensities and forces, into a field of *meaning*. Unconscious phantasy is a hybrid concept, between psyche and body, inside and outside, word and feeling.

Susan Isaacs' text (1952/1989) on the nature and function of phantasy remains an important reference today. It was presented to the British Psychoanalytic Society during the Freud–Klein controversy (1941–1945), during which there was heated debate over whether Kleinian theories diverted from Freudian thought. This controversy foregrounded a struggle for institutional power among young, aspiring psychoanalysts – and it generated excellent intellectual production, such as Isaacs'.

Isaacs (1952/1982, p. 127) asserts that "(…) phantasies are the primary contents of unconscious mental processes" (p. 82);[2] and that "Unconscious phantasies are primarily about bodies, and represent instinctual aims towards objects" (p. 112).

Ogden (2012) returned to Isaacs' work after many decades and wrote an instigating piece proposing that the understanding of unconscious phantasy precedes, in some respects, Bion's (1962/2014) theory of thinking.

Following Bion's understanding of unconscious phantasy, analysts clearly understood that the capacity for thought is born out of the sensory world of emotional experience, anchored in bodily sensation. In the 1943 version of the text,[3] Isaacs (1943/1998, p. 243) argues: "The primary content of all mental processes are unconscious phantasies. Such phantasies are the basis of all unconscious and conscious thought processes". We know, from Isaacs and even more clearly from Bion, that phantasy is proto-thought; it is a primitive, emotional, and sensory experience that over time organizes and takes shape, maintaining a continuity – or better, an invariance – that connects unconscious thought, or proto-thought, to more abstract thought.

Unconscious phantasies are, then, the psychic representatives of stimuli such as hunger, thirst, cold and heat, sensations, desires, bodily processes like feeding and excretion, as well as plans, projects, ideas, and ideals. To this we might also add ways of speaking and walking, bodily posture, ways of dealing with time (punctuality and procrastination) and money (frugality or lavishness) – all of which are connected to conflicts with authority, being fundamentally based in an unconscious phantasy, as are phobias, hysterical conversions and obsessive rituals.

In short, "Nothing that occurs in the body and in the mind ceases to be, in some way, associated to this unconscious and creative act of phantasy" (Figueiredo, 2009, p. 25).

Unconscious phantasy is, therefore, the capacity to create scenes, situations, and theories out of all lived experience, giving meaning and value to everything that happens. We can say that an infant's first discoveries of the world – in the oral and anal stages – happen by devouring and grasping at objects, the archaic modes of appropriating the world for oneself. We can trace a line of continuity from the baby's – and even the foetus's – act of *grasping* to the adult's more abstract cognitive act of *comprehending*. Here the English language illustrates the continuity: the verb "to grasp" can mean both "to grab with one's hands" and "to understand".

When an analyst interprets, they develop an attention that fluctuates between the bodily and the psychic; in other words, they imagine the psyche with the body as a backdrop. Unconscious phantasies, in their hybridity, are able to mediate between such heterogenous dimensions as affects, words, and bodily sensation. This makes it possible to translate a moral conflict, for example, into bodily, primitive, and infantile terms. These transpositions of meaning help the patient to make the analyst's interpretation more *carnal*, which in turn becomes more nuanced, forming an insight out of an emotional experience, and thus psychic change might occur. These processes of transposition accomplished by interpretation – between body and psyche, outside and inside, past and present – are shifts in meaning made possible through transference, thanks to the mediating mobility of unconscious phantasy.

To conclude these considerations, we can assert, alongside Figueiredo (2009), that there are more or less pathological ways of dealing with unconscious phantasy. Those mechanisms that are closer to an idea of "health" involve admitting, expressing, and symbolizing the most archaic phantasies, in the same way that pathology seeks to repress them and uses more radical defence mechanisms against them, such as denial, disavowal, and splitting.

Through the analytic process, one hopes to process and transform unconscious phantasies. One must share their most archaic and omnipotent phantasies with another person in order to deal with them; in the early stages of life, with the mother and other carers, and later in life, with the analyst. The analytic project seeks to provide ample space for the expression of unconscious phantasies, in the hopes of diminishing their omnipotence and generating a growing process of symbolization. The incessant work of collecting and symbolizing unconscious phantasies can lead to a significant expansion of the capacity to think and feel.

Having to hand a concept like unconscious phantasy, in its many articulations and levels of development, as a concept that crosses somatic and psychic realities, allows the analyst to listen to *representations* and at the same time open themselves up to a new way of listening to the *unrepresentable* and the *unconscious memories of the body*. Through this concept, it is possible to travel creatively between Freud's first and second topographies, articulating the clinic of representation and the clinic of instincts.

Notes

1 An idea articulated in Figueiredo (2006).
2 Phantasy's intermediary position between body and psyche is close to the notion of imaginative elaboration of bodily functions, proposed by Winnicott, too, in the 1950s.
3 There are two versions of Susan Isaacs' text, the 1943 original presented during the controversy and a revised version published in 1952.

References

Bion, R. W. (1959/2014). On arrogance. In: *The complete works of W. R. Bion*. London: Karnac.

Bion, R. W. (1962/2014). Learning from experience. In: *The complete works of W. R. Bion*. London: Karnac.

Cintra, E. M. U. and Figueiredo L. C. (2004). *Melanie Klein: Estilo e pensamento*. (Free translation: Melanie Klein: Style and thoughts). São Paulo: Escuta.

Figueiredo, L. C. (2009). A clínica psicanalítica a partir de Melanie Klein. O que isso pode significar? In: *As diversas faces do cuidar*. (Free translation: The various facets of care – new essays in contemporary psychoanalysis). São Paulo: Escuta.

Freud, S. (1923/2024). The ego and the id. In: *The revised standard edition of the complete psychological works of Sigmund Freud*. London: Rowman & Littlefield (original translation by James Strachey and revised, supplemented and edited by Mark Solms).

Isaacs, S. (1943/1991). The nature and function of phantasy. In: *The Freud-Klein controversies 1941–1945* (edited by Pearl King and Riccardo Steiner). London: Routledge.

Isaacs, S. and others (1952/1989). The nature and function of phantasy. In: *Developments of psychoanalysis*. London: Karnac.

Ogden, T. H. (2012). Reading Susan Isaacs: Toward a radically revised theory of thinking. In: *Creative readings*. London; New York: Routledge.

5 The archaic in Klein

Elisa Maria de Ulhôa Cintra and
Marina F. R. Ribeiro

At the heart of the Kleinian legacy is its language. Its constant reference to bodily fluids and organs brings us directly in touch with the concrete and corporeal dimension of infantile phantasy. And perhaps it is this very aspect that might at first provoke a rejection of Kleinian ideas, frightening not just the lay reader but other psychoanalysts.

Indeed, many psychoanalysts confess to having been shocked when they first read Melanie Klein. They recognize, however, that it was Klein who taught us to find the words to precisely articulate the child's psychic universe, a dimension that lives on in adult life. As adults, we are often confronted with the child's omnipotence, their rage, their wrath, their despair and helplessness, their conflicts in the face of good and bad objects. It is so difficult to know how to deal with our inner child: at times we spoil them too much, at others we unfairly pick on them. That is, rather than harassing or overly protecting our inner child, we must give them a voice; we must listen to them.

So, in order to read Klein and fully grasp her ideas, it is especially important to follow an approach that remains vital today: observe how children play; how they care for or seek to possess their objects of love and hate; how their desire to control, hurt, and damage their toys and their real or imaginary friends manifests; how they enact their needs, fears, and anxieties, their pleasure in dominating others; how in doing so they exercise their power or reveal the instinct to deny separation from their loved ones.

For Klein, the oral, anal, urethral, and phallic dimensions of child sexuality continue to manifest over the span of a lifetime, like a lower layer or substratum of adult eroticism. They continue to express themselves diversely through the phantasies of devouring, expelling, constricting, controlling, or submitting.

Through her personal and clinical observation of play and the psychic life of children and babies, Klein guides us to the *archaic psychic dimension*, and in doing so contributed to an understanding of the deepest and most primitive workings of the unconscious. Indeed, the unconscious demands that the psychoanalyst have an analytic mode of listening and a capacity for metaphor. This brings us to one of Klein's central preoccupations: the emotional

DOI: 10.4324/9781003583035-6

experience of the analyst and the patient during the session, which, alongside *learning from experience*, were ideas extensively developed by Bion[1] and Winnicott and, later, by Thomas Ogden, Christopher Bollas, and Antonino Ferro, to name a few.

There is, however, a tricky paradox at the heart of all emotional experience: there is, on the one hand, the need to be in touch with raw emotions and their brutal and violent states, that reveal the archaic need to appropriate the other in order to possess them; and, on the other, the need to be free from and to free the other, separating oneself from the infantile unconscious and standing alone. This is the paradox of the simultaneous desire to be loved and recognized, and the desire to be free; and at the same time obey the ethical duty to care for and truly see the other. in their singularity.

We can say, then, that the enigma of love and its violent possessiveness is at the heart of Klein's thought. Klein was sensitive, more than any other analyst, to the paradox, as articulated by Freud, that we are like porcupines, always eager to experience love, moved by what he called *Sensucht*, a voracious longing to love and be loved, a desire for intimacy; and, at the same time, once we are close enough to the other, out come the sharp spines and we discover the dark side of human nature, its violence and possessiveness. "Homo homini lupus", says Freud (1930/2024, p. 100), recalling Hobbes' famous words.[2] This is our almost irreducible violence, our infantile need to possess and enslave the other.

Humans are characterized by the need to feel secure, loved, and recognized on the one hand, and a desire to have power and control over loved and hated ones on the other. When these needs and desires are frustrated, they lead to rage, wrath, and violence. This is a bitterly pessimist point of agreement between Freud in *Civilisation and its Discontents* and Klein's emphasis on the destructive dimensions of the primitive mind. Psychoanalysts, however, hope that it might be possible to reduce and transform a part of these hostile tendency, and it is this hope to which they dedicate their work.

The primordial relationship to the mother and the "Oedipal situation"

Decipher me, or I will devour you.

(Tebas' sphinx, *Oedipus Rex*)

The Hungarian psychoanalyst Ferenczi (1924/1938) used the term "amphimixis" to articulate the polymorphous nature of child sexuality – the simultaneous presence of all erotic forms, i.e., the oral, anal, urethral, phallic, sadistic, fetishist, and so on.[3]

Inspired by Ferenczi, Melanie Klein understood that, in the unconscious and archaic realm, there is a certain infiltration of eroticisms, each coloring the other, as if orality transmitted something of its phantasy of devouring and consuming to the anal dimension; and anality, with its connection to muscularity and the domination instinct, transmitted to the oral scope something of its logic, which we can summarize in the terms "retain-expel", "approach-retreat". This formulation led Klein to conceive of a similar idea, that dual and triangular relationships are not mutually exclusive, but can coexist. In this way the separation between stages becomes less clear and recalls the Freudian metaphor of a landscape in which different kinds of vegetation grow and mingle.

It was Melanie Klein, though, who, before any other analyst after Freud, intuited the existence of an incipient Oedipal triangle from the first months of life. Though the first object relations are predominantly dual and oral, with very little differentiation between mother and baby, the first acknowledgement of difference, of alterity, begins to emerge very early on. Klein thought that the "bad breast", or the unpleasant sensations attributed to the mother or to the maternal environment, could serve as the *third element* of an incipient Oedipal triangle.

With her clinical intuition, Klein highlighted the importance of the body and the baby's interaction with the mother's body in primitive forms. What is now considered intrinsic to psychoanalytic investigations was, in the 1920s and 1930s, seen as extremely bold and thus misunderstood.

Eventually, however, Klein's followers developed this perspective, and it entered the mainstream. In the 1950s and 1960s, Winnicott and Bion investigated the beginnings of psychic life based on this primordial relationship with the mother. Winnicott developed the concepts of the holding environment (1958/1990), the good-enough mother (1957/1964), and primary maternal preoccupation (1958/1990); and Bion (1962/2014) used the mother–baby model to structure his theory of thinking.

In early life, the baby does not perceive the mother as separate from their own body; however, between the fourth and sixth month of life, when babies begin to wean, the frequent absence of the mother makes it possible to perceive her as a separate figure. In other words, when the experience of the mother's absence occurs, the archaic Oedipus complex begins (Klein, 1928/1960). The mother's *absence* creates a new understanding of her *presence*, which now stands out and can be discerned outside the symbiotic union. The experience of the mother's absence makes the father or other caregivers become more perceptible, precisely because of the strangeness created when they appear in the mother's place.

We can better understand the precocity of the Oedipal triangulation from this excerpt from a book by Cintra and Figueiredo (2004, p. 28):

> The characters that feature in this early Oedipal triangle or drama are **the child**—whose ego begins to form more distinctly at the very moment they can perceive the mother as a whole object—**the mother**, they begin to recognize, and **the stranger**, whose existence is painfully discovered precisely because it marks the mother's absence.

From this perspective, the father is the first *familiar stranger*. The primary object for both boys and girls is the mother, and on the emotional horizon of the child-and-their-mother, the father appears immediately after the infant's early perception of the mother as an "other" (a whole object). The father is, initially, the horizon into which the mother has disappeared. Put differently, the father is first experienced as a stranger – he is still the non-mother.

The precocity of the Oedipal triangulation is a hallmark of Klein's thought (1928/1960). The baby is driven by the oral frustration imposed by the mother during weaning to turn toward other sources of satisfaction, whereupon they encounter the father. This movement occurs concurrently with the depressive position, a concept that Klein would go on to articulate in 1935 and 1945, as we will explain later. Petot (1979/1982) states that the ego "flees and distributes"; that is, it flees from frustration and distributes its investments beyond the primary object.

Therefore, the state of fusion and undifferentiation in early life does not last long; the frustration of the idyllic primary object (the mother) brings forth the non-mother, from whence the father, and after him the world, come into view. Pain, discomfort, the father – these are the carriers of triangularity that appear on the external horizon of the original dyad between mother and baby. The result is disjunction; indeed, at any age, there is always a certain disjunction between the subject and their objects. It is from this disjunction that babies and adults imagine the so-called primal scene. This unconscious phantasy, inscribed in the psyche from the beginning of life, is easier to understand if we assume that at the instant that the mother's plenitude is ruptured and is suddenly no longer there, plenitude is projected outward to an imaginary place where supposedly it might happen instead. It is this outward movement that creates the primal scene – a nearly inconceivable feast of pleasure – where plenitude, the pain linked to the loss of plenitude, the nostalgia of this loss, and the desire to reclaim it are simultaneous.

In this fictitious place, the subject comes to occupy the position of the excluded third, a position necessary for them to be able to imagine themselves from the outside as an object and to develop the capacity to think and feel, as we will further clarify below.

Klein called this original triangularity the "Oedipal situation" (1928), associating it with the multitude of affects that interrupt the initial experience of satisfaction. Gratification continues to be desired but is displaced: it now belongs to the realm of memory, nostalgia, and the incessant search to attain it again in some future moment; that is, it has been transferred to the realm of phantasy and, later, of thought.

For Klein (1928/1960a, 1932/1960b, and 1935/1975), before entering the Oedipus complex proper, as described by Freud, the child experiences the "Oedipal situation", the realization that the mother has other sources of pleasure. This occurs when the mother is absent or fails, and the child is overwhelmed with questions: Where did she go? Who is she with now? This imaginary and indistinct situation anticipates the entry into the Oedipus complex proper, between three and five years of age.

As Figueiredo (2009, p. 41) states, "In this sense, there is an early and incipient triangular situation, somewhat indistinct, as the limit of bliss". Bliss and the primary idyll need to find a boundary, both in reality and in phantasy. In reality, the father and other objects functioning as the third need to support and enable the dual relationship between the second – the mother – and the first – the baby – who are involved in a mutual narcissistic primordial phantasy of omnipotence.

The dual relationship, no matter how compelling and attractive, generates considerable anxiety: the simultaneous desire for and fear of diving in and losing oneself in the other. The presence of the father and other "thirds" is supportive for the mother, enabling her in turn to support the baby; and at the same time, it sets a limit on the maternal tendency to merge with the baby and exert absolute control over them. In other words, the father protects the mother from the anxiety of engulfment.

Perhaps Klein's most enriching contribution to the understanding of the "crossing and dissolution of the Oedipus complex" was her likening it to a process of mourning and separation, building upon existing psychoanalytic reflection on mourning and melancholia, dating back to 1915. In this way, it became possible to conceive of an Oedipal crossing in accordance with a healthy process of mourning; and, on the other end of the spectrum, cases of misguided crossings are seen to approach the conditions of melancholia, paranoia, and schizophrenia.

At the same time, Klein's strategy of consistently thinking in terms of "situations" and "positions", which group anxieties and defences, offered her a more flexible path. This approach allowed her to comprehend the infinite combinations and configurations that each child creates to manage their needs, demands, desires, defences, and anxieties, in their integration into the family world and their construction of a place in the world.

This way of thinking in terms of anxieties, defences, and modes of object relations enabled Klein to discern, construct, and deconstruct the formative elements of the Oedipus complex retrospectively as if they were building blocks, beginning with the creation and destruction of different forms of the Oedipal situation during weaning.

The Oedipal situation can then develop in the child in either a more defensive or structuring manner; in the latter case, it becomes possible to deconstruct primary narcissism and enter a process of symbolization. In truth, Klein does not frequently refer to primary narcissism as Freud conceived of it; she believed that narcissism was not absolute, for it was always accompanied by object relations from very early life. What we call "primary narcissism" here corresponds in Klein's thinking to the schizoid-paranoid position and the "early stages of Oedipus conflict" (Klein, 1928, 1932). Instead of primary narcissism, the *archaic* in Klein is better expressed as the primary *states of a narcissistic omnipotence*.

The fundamental question that remains decisive across all schools of psychoanalysis is: "How does one emerge from narcissistic omnipotence and the omnipotent, combined, and confused figures as they are arranged in unconscious phantasy?" (Figueiredo, 2009, p. 42).

In Kleinian terms, a sign that we are in the early stages of the Oedipal conflict is the presence of the "combined parental figure", which merge the father and mother into a relationship that absolutely excludes everything and everyone. This relationship is fantasized according to a sadistic, violent, intense, and chaotic dynamic, corresponding to the excessive nature of oral, anal, and urethral sexuality, along with muscular eroticism in its earliest forms.

So, when the child feels excluded by this so-called combined parental figure, they feel intense pain and hatred towards the parental couple, conceiving of them as idealized good or bad objects.

The Brazilian film *City of God* (2002), directed by Fernando Meirelles and Kátia Lund, depicts an extremely violent enactment of the kinds of violence that can arise from this type of phantasy. A boy raised in a dysfunctional environment invades a motel and shoots all the couples inside. To the boy, the parental couple appears to celebrate an inconceivable pleasure, and he experiences this as a radical exclusion. Adult sexuality seems enigmatic, exclusionary, and violent because it embodies the child's own violent reaction against it. To counteract the feeling of exclusion from adult sexuality, which in the scene represents all the other exclusions the boy has faced, the only option left is to commit the most radical act of destruction.

Regarding this fear of adult sexuality, Figueiredo highlights: "In the fantasized primal scene, the omnipotent object is created—a protector who is both all-encompassing and terrifying, possessing all attributes and capacities, the mother's interior with an internal penis" (2009, p. 42). This autoerotic and self-sufficient object gathers and unites the most intense phantasies of pleasure, violence, and power. The idea of the all-powerful "combined parents" is Klein's way of expressing this phantasy.

For this phantasy to arise, the child need not witness a sadomasochistic or other sexual relationship; it may arise simply from living with a narcissistic and autoerotic mother. Sometimes the presence of a radically and violently failing environment is enough to generate the phantasy of the combined parents in a baby who feels helpless.

It is worth pointing out that any monstrous figure that represents ideals of power and excellence and threats of exclusion, can constitute the figure of the "combined parents". Other instigating experiences might include the figure of a dictator or authoritarian societies. These radical environments create an idealized "good" in leaders and dominant social groups, necessarily vilifying and excluding another social group, as we have seen before the genocides of the 20th and 21st centuries.

What seems to lend these social orders credibility is their offer of absolute protection to their followers, who desire this protection intensely, but in exchange for radical obedience, as seen in Islamist *jihad*. The Kleinian archaic superego behaves according to similar stipulations, with its violent injunctions, recriminations, and deprecations.

Triangularity brings about moderation. The relationship between dictator and an ordinary person is a dual one, where the former is hyper-powerful, and the latter is hyper-weak. There is no mediation in this dynamic, and so the person is at risk of being quashed. This danger is reflected on a smaller scale in archaic forms of an indistinct *triangularity*, in which the figures of the second and third are still threateningly amalgamated, casting a shadow over the self.

The paranoid-schizoid organizes this triangularity by phantasizing about the mother and father being either strictly good or strictly bad – that is, the parental figures are dissociated. Various dual relationships can then be created, such as idealizing the mother to escape a "bad" father, or the opposite. In these defensive configurations, triangulation does not appear clearly. Kleinians believe that the depressive position, the polarities of good and bad can be integrated, and one is able to exit the realm of extremes.

Thus, for the Oedipus complex to be resolved, the child must perceive the maternal and paternal figures as ambivalent, that is, good *and* bad, and be able to differentiate between a relationship of tender alliance and one of eroticism. The subject must relinquish incestuous phantasies – the desire to form an elective and idealized relationship with the mother or father by eliminating the rival – and enter mechanisms of filiation instead, experiencing relative states of discrimination, union, and separation.

As Freud argues, if the child works through several depressive positions within the first five years of life, they will have mastered the most important elaboration of the Oedipus complex. As a result, the child can conceive of a benign parental couple, united by tenderness and eroticism and differentiated from one other, joining and separating non-violently. At the same time, the father and mother exclude the children from the erotic relationship and include them in the parental alliance that provides support and nurturing. This the introjected "good object", which affects future emotional relationships in adult life, teaching us to navigate the demands of intimacy and freedom in friendships and sexual and loving relationships.

The child must learn to deal with the difference between sexual relations and tender intimacy, moving from an absolute dependence on their parents to a relative dependence. This becomes necessary with future partners, allowing for freedom within attachments. The child must be able to exclude the other at certain moments and allow themselves to be excluded by the loved one, so that individual freedoms can be preserved and there is a constant moderation of the desires to dominate and to be dominated, which do not completely disappear in adult sexuality but must be transformed and sublimated.

The good object, introjected as a non-combined parental couple, also allows the archaic anxieties of separation and engulfment, with their potential threat of annihilation, to be transformed into castration anxiety and guilt, which are more easily processed. This makes non-manic reparation possible, as milder anxieties can be transformed into acts of true reparation by learning to be alone, to care, and to allow oneself to be cared for, and to engage in the multiplicity of cultural life.

Accepting the presence of a third – the so-called "other of the other", meaning the other of the primary object – is crucial to working through the depressive position. Acceptance of this presence teaches the advantages of occupying the position of the third in a relationship. Being the child excluded from parental sexuality is the foundation of the capacity for thought: thought, the act of observing and symbolizing, can only be established if one occupies the position of the third. It is in the absence of satisfaction and the absence of the object that the processes of representation and thought can begin. It is successive separations and their resulting enigmas that give rise to the child's questions – "Where do babies come from? What are they made of? Where was I before I was born?" – and the need to develop cognitive and self-reflective abilities to deal with the mysteries of the world.

The subject-in-the-making thus becomes both a subject who wants to know the world and an object to be known by themselves and by others. They need to move in and out of emotional relationships through the position of the third, which allows them to circulate among various places – stepping out of the protagonist's place and returning to it at alternate moments to see from afar, with perspective, and to see themselves from the outside, through the eyes of others and through their own gaze, which they identify with the gaze of others.

Thus, it is the occupied position of the third that unleashes the "epistemophilic instinct", strengthening the K (knowledge) link, which Bion (1962/2014) considers to be of great importance as a form of mediation and transformation of the L (love) and H (hate) links.

Figueiredo (2009, p. 44) articulates it thus: "In the absence of triangulation, knowledge and thought are inhibited, and love and hate relationships prevail without moderation".

The transformation of the Oedipus complex into a *situation* allowed Klein to playfully and flexibly see this complex from multiple angles. The fluidity of the Oedipal situation is also one of the precursors to the notion of the paternal *function*. By thinking in terms of *positions* – paranoid-schizoid and depressive – it becomes easier to conceive of roles occupied by characters during the formation of the psychic subject, transforming the concrete characters – the father, the mother – into occupiable *positions*. This way of conceptualizing the Oedipus complex sets it into motion, instead of becoming a rigid structure with fixed characters.

To move beyond primary narcissism – a decisive issue stated a few pages back – and to ensure the healthy evolution of the Oedipal situation, the paternal function must be satisfactorily established. But what does this mean?

The paternal function depends on the child effectively occupying the third position and the mother accepting she must leave the place of original symbiosis to become an "interrupted" mother. This is the process we might call the healthy evolution of the Oedipal situation, starting from the time of weaning, before the Oedipus complex fully manifests.

When the paternal function is not well established, the child may feel entirely excluded from the parental couple or, conversely, included in a violent and confusing way, which often occurs in borderline pathologies. In response to these situations, one might attempt a defensive strategy by constructing "Psychic Retreats" (Steiner, 1993), which protect the subject from both exclusion and overly intense inclusion.

Other forms of neurotic Oedipal situations include the development of excessive rivalries, jealousy, and envy, or, as a counter to this excessive turbulence, becoming of indifferent to and depreciative of parents and peers. Fantasies may arise, such as "my mother loves me more than she loves my father", leading to great instability, homicidal fantasies, or manic reparations. This is what happens in the case of a visible Oedipus complex, as described by Britton (1998).

To avoid these outcomes, which we consider more pathological, an effective occupation of the third position associated with the paternal function is necessary. During the period of mother–baby symbiosis, the paternal function is to protect and contain the dyad in a non-invasive way; it is, therefore, about enabling symbiosis. In the first months after birth, the father must also draw the mother's libido toward him so that she can exit the narcissistic monad and experience moments of freedom from the maternal function, reclaiming herself as a person. This function can be fulfilled by somebody with whom the woman has a significant relationship or by any other interest that strongly attracts her: "There needs to be erotic investment by her and in her so that the mother is revitalized and the third is legitimised" (Figueiredo, 2009, p. 47).

In other words, the mother must find revitalization and eroticism outside the narcissistic unit so she can return to the baby with renewed energy. The presence of the father is important to dislodge unconscious fantasies of remaining forever in a dual-narcissistic relationship; his presence initiates the process of deconstructing primary narcissism. As the child grows, they will then encounter a parental couple that excludes and includes them in a variety of ways. This makes it possible for the child to introject a *good object*, a viable alternative to the fantasies of absolute symbiotic union. The child must find an object of interest alternative to the mother (like a teddy-bear), where they can relinquish all-encompassing primary narcissism. This object of interest then functions as a point of reference for freer relationships of love, hate, and knowledge.

Both Bion and Winnicott argue strongly that parental relationships characterized by trust strongly contribute to mental health. These kinds of relationship allow Oedipal anxieties to be worked through, particularly when the father does not discredit the mother, and the mother does not belittle the father. Both can then create an atmosphere of trust and validation for the child, thus at least in part reducing envy, rivalry, and jealousy. The evolutionary processes of moving beyond primary narcissism and working through the Oedipus complex consequently influence emotional, cognitive, ethical, and sensorial development.

But what about in the analytic practice, where can we discern the third position? The third can be discerned through the setting of the analysis, how it is handled, and the interpretations performed by the analyst; these are the elements of the "framing structure" (Green, 2001, p. 77). They create a boundary that delineates what transpires in the relationship with the patient, such as the fundamental rule "say whatever comes to mind", the scheduling, and the cost of the session. When the analyst remains faithful to their therapeutic project, theoretical convictions, and internal objects – those with whom they learned their craft, their own analyst, supervisors, and the therapeutic community to which they belong – these entities fulfil the role of the third in their relationship with the patient.

The analyst can thus occupy various positions: they are the subject of countertransference, the object of the patient's transference, while still maintaining the place of observer of the scene unfolding in the analysis. They need to occupy the place of the first, the subject, and the place of the second, the object, but their activity depends on being able to occupy the place of the third, thus maintaining a reserved position as one who reflects on what is being experienced.

Figueiredo (2009, p. 50) highlights: "Any interpretation, regardless of its specific content, attests to the independence, autonomy, and thinking capacity of the analyst [...] Any interpretation establishes a new angle in the relationship, a vertex of triangulation". This is what leads some patients to reject the analyst's interpretation, claiming to have already noticed or understood what the analyst suggests. The analysand transfers the difficulty they feel in admitting the new, which belongs to this third place that lies outside their relationship to the known, to the analysis itself.

Caper (1999), inspired by Klein, Bion, and Britton, advises the analyst to maintain a "mind of their own", staying true to their internal objects and to psychoanalytic theory itself, so that they can uphold their position as a third alongside the patient and the patient's convictions.

In Figueiredo's words, sometimes "the analyst must be available for a close and almost fusion-like relationship; but for this to become therapeutic, the place of the third element must be occupied, whether by the setting, the analyst's internal objects, or a supervisor" (2009, p. 50).

This proper occupation of the third place, in the sense of one who can always disentangle themselves from passionate emotions and convictions, is a prerequisite for the therapeutic effect of psychoanalysis.

Finally, we can ask ourselves: what are the consequences of Kleinian thought for psychoanalytic practice in its later development? Still inspired by Figueiredo (2009), we consider that Bion's clinical approach (1962, 1965, 1970) greatly benefited from Klein's theoretical perspective, creating three clinical models: a clinic of containment, a clinic of confrontation, and a clinic of emptiness.

The clinic of containment proposes that the analyst can receive and contain the patient's unconscious phantasies, transforming them through the analyst's own *rêverie*. Bion discusses the notions of "container and contained", of "beta-elements" and "alpha-function".

The second clinic – the clinic of confrontation – proposes working on the patient's life of phantasies. Confronting the patient does not mean imposing one's model of truth and reality on them; it means inviting them to untangle their phantasies, which are repressed or split, to create a working field together within this terrain, aiming to elucidate the conflicts between the emotional aspects that seek expression and the defences that clash with them.

The third clinic is an invitation to venture into the silence and void of images, beyond preconceived ideas, towards the unexpected and the unknown. The analyst must then develop a negative capability – listening without memory, without desire, without a too-rapid prior understanding (Bion, 1970), to free themselves from their personal and theoretical preconceptions and develop a "pure, receptive, anticipatory, poetic, and creative capacity to expect the unexpected" (Figueiredo, 2009, p. 49).

The archaic anguishes or psychotic anxieties

Before Klein, Freud associated anxiety with unsatisfied libido, especially in his first theory of anxiety. Freud considered the quantitative, rather than qualitative, aspect of anxiety; that is, he was more concerned with the intensity of anxiety than with the phantasies associated with it. Gradually, he became interested in phantasies and the archaic situations of angst and danger (Freud, 1926). Anxiety came to be seen as the affect released in anticipation of a previously experienced dangerous situation, such as the danger of leaving intrauterine life at birth.

Otto Rank believed that all anxiety was the reliving of the trauma of birth. Freud (1926), however, understood the metaphor of birth as a general model for the passage from a state of homeostasis to an unknown state; he debated with Rank over the generalizability of this model, arguing that situations of danger and anxiety change according to the stage of life.

In 1926, Freud accepted the idea of birth trauma as the prototype of anxiety, considering that this first form would later be re-signified through the various stages of sexual libido – oral, anal, urethral, sadistic-oral, sadistic-anal, sadistic-urethral – which would give new configurations to the feared dangerous situation. In the phallic phase and the Oedipus complex, original anxiety would appear in the form of castration anxiety.

In the article "Inhibitions, Symptoms and Anxiety", Freud (1926) clearly spoke of archaic situations of anxiety or danger. The article inspired Melanie Klein (1928) to think about archaic anxieties based on this model, that is, focusing on identifying the dangerous situation implicit in the anxiety. Interestingly, Klein began to write about the Oedipal situation around the same time Freud wrote of these dangerous situations.

From the beginning of her clinical work, Klein observed that children's play led to many phantasies and dramatic enactments involving cruelty and aggression, followed by a severe form of remorse and guilt. Klein was always struck by the violence and sadism present in children's phantasies and the fear of retribution and the return of the most aggressive aspects of these phantasies upon themselves. The fear of being annihilated, the anxious guilt of having harmed or damaged, inhibited aggressive phantasies and, consequently, the epistemophilic instinct, the desire to know – a situation that generated inhibitions and learning difficulties observed by Klein in young children.

For Klein, the main instinctual conflict is one between aggression (death drive) and remorse (which comes from the life drive, libido, and love). Archaic or psychotic anxieties create a vicious cycle that is self-perpetuating. Aggression generates fear, which in turn generates more aggression.

In "A Contribution to the Psychogenesis of Manic-Depressive States" (1935), Klein developed the theory of the depressive position and proposed that the main archaic anxiety was the fear of losing the mother or caregiver and its internal representative, the so-called "internal good object".

In her 1932 book *The Psychoanalysis of Children*, Klein argued for the existence of two types of archaic anxieties: one more characteristic of the depressive position, with its tone of guilt and the impression of having damaged the object and the relationship with it, which includes a certain concern for the object's fate; and another with a more persecutory and paranoid tone, involving the fear of being annihilated by the object, with a focus on the damage that the ego may suffer.

In "Notes on Some Schizoid Mechanisms" (1946) Melanie Klein more clearly defined the theory of persecutory anxiety, which is the fear of ego annihilation and is more self-referential than depressive anxiety. Its axis is more narcissistic, whereas the depressive position is more outward facing. We could translate persecutory anxiety in a simplified way as the following example: "I fear that my 'I' will be destroyed".

From the beginning, when faced with a child, Melanie Klein considered it important to interpret the most urgent anxieties and defences in the material presented by the child through play. She began to investigate the real and imagined situations of danger and anxiety in children. She began with Freud's idea that the child's main archaic anxiety is the loss of the beloved and protective figure (the mother, the father, the "parental figure", the caregiver), for whom the child feels a very strong desire, which creates a situation of greater danger in moments of need and dependence on parental help. She found that infantile love is extremely intense. Since parents and caregivers are inevitably subject to various types of failures and absences when the child needs them, this archaic situation can generate phantasies of attack on the mother's body, which express the aggressions born out of unrequited love and, spontaneously, from the death instinct.

Children then have aggressive and libidinal instincts to steal everything good the mother has, to definitively appropriate everything they need from the mother's body. Primitive love is violent, as it seeks to suck, incorporate, control, and be exclusive. The fear that the mother will harm them is, then, mostly the return of a sadistic phantasy. The paranoid phantasy that the mother will attack, kill, rob, or abandon them, and imagine the mother taking revenge for the insatiability of infantile love.

Later, depressive anxieties also arise, as the child fears that the mother, feeling abandoned and ruined by the child's excessive demands, might die. The more furious or damaged the parents are, the more they are transformed into internal persecutors; the child unleashes all their sadistic weapons to destroy them; in this way, the phantasized parents become all-powerful and threaten to destroy the sadistic child. These archaic *imagos* are, in part, the effect of the child's own violence and sadism, generating the vicious cycle of paranoia. In such cases, anxiety can become so intense that Klein began referring to it as psychotic anxiety (1932).

Psychotic anxieties are those that have not yet been worked through by the ego and have not been symbolized, hence why they are intense, paralyze the ego, and have aspects of paranoia. They suggest that the person may be feeling a terrifying fear of having committed an act of great destruction. These phantasies are affectively supercharged and omnipotent. If the person feels guilt over the destruction committed, a fragile sense of identification with the dead or injured person may emerge. Psychotic anxieties are, like neurotic anxieties, those that do not yet have a face, name, or figure; that is, they cannot be thought of. They are in a raw state and follow an absolute "all or nothing" regime, immediately, without mediation or consideration for the complexity of psychic phenomena. They provoke states of symbolic abolition, major acting out, and delinquency.

Paranoid or persecutory anxiety, that is, the pure panic of receiving retribution for everything done to the other (even if only in imagination), changes significantly with the entry into the depressive position, when the attacked object can no longer be seen as a purely bad object but becomes a complex mixture of good and bad.

Faced with depressive anxieties, a serious fear for the object arises, and no longer only for the destruction of the self, as when persecutory anxieties predominate. An intense fear of having damaged the good object emerges, along with the beginnings of a sense of responsibility, care, and guilt.

However, if guilt becomes overwhelming, it transforms into persecutory feelings, leading to a regression to the previous position, giving rise to a desperate sense that the damage is irreparable. This is the archaic anxiety in its depressive state, which involves crying, lamentation, desperate sorrow, and fear of having already destroyed and ruined without any possible solution. Depressive anxiety is characterized by the fear for the loved object, for the continuity of the relationship of love and care towards it.

The desperate lament, the sorrow for the loved and irreparably lost object, can be softened by an increase in libido, by loving feelings that counteract sadism, thereby enhancing the importance of the good internal objects and the confidence in the reparative power of love.

We have thus seen that Melanie Klein proposed the theory of positions to explain how subjects articulate their defences, construct their identifications, direct themselves towards their objects, relate to them, and either navigate or are overwhelmed by their archaic anxieties.

Notes

1 The term "emotional experience" appears constantly in Bion's work (1962), indicating that the transformative aspect of analysis lies in the emotional experience lived between analyst and analysand.
2 A free translation would be "Man is wolf to man".
3 "The sexual development of the individual culminates, according to the Drei Abhandlungen, in the supersession by the primacy of the genital zone of the hitherto active autoerotisms ... and of the previous organizations of sexuality, whereby the erotisms and the stages of organization which have been thus transcended are retained in the final genital organization as mechanisms of fore-pleasure" (Ferenczi, 1924/1938, p. 9).

References

Bion, W. R. (1962/2014). Learning from experience. In: *The complete works of W. R. Bion*. London: Karnac. Edited by Chris Mawson and editorial consultancy by Francesca Bion.

Bion, W. R. (1965/2014). Transformations: Change from learning to growth. In: *The complete works of W. R. Bion*. London: Karnac. Edited by Chris Mawson.

Bion, W. R. (1970/2014). Attention and interpretation: A scientific approach to insight in psychoanalysis and groups. In: *The complete works of W. R. Bion*. London: Karnac. Edited by Chris Mawson and editorial consultancy by Francesca Bion.

Britton, R. (1998). *Belief and imagination*. London; New York: Routledge.

Caper, R. (1999). *A mind of one's own – a Kleinian view of self and object*. New York: Routledge.

Cintra, E. M. U. and Figueiredo, L. C. (2004). *Melanie Klein: Estilo e pensamento*. São Paulo: Escuta. (translation: Melanie Klein: Style and Thoughts).

Ferenczi, S. (1924/1938). *Thalassa: A theory of genitality*. New York: The Psychoanalytic Quarterly. Translated by Henry Alden Bunker.

Figueiredo, L. C. (2009). *As diversas faces do cuidar – novos ensaios de psicanálise contemporânea*. São Paulo: Escuta. (translation: The Various Faces of Caring – New Essays on Contemporary Psychoanalysis).

Freud, S. (1926/1959). *Inhibitions, symptoms and anxiety*. New York; London: W. W. Norton and Company. Translated by Alix Strachey, revised and edited by James Strachey.

Freud, S. (1930/2024). Civilization and its discontents. In: *The revised standard edition of the complete psychological works of Sigmund Freud*. Maryland: Rowman & Littlefield. Translation by Joan Riviere and edited by Ernest Jones.

Green, A. (2001). *Life narcissism, death narcissism*. London: Free Association Books.

Klein, M. (1928/1960a). Early stages of the Oedipus conflict and of super-ego formation. In: *The psychoanalysis of children*. New York: Grove Press.

Klein, M. (1932/1960b). The effects of early anxiety-situations on the sexual development of the girl. In: *The psychoanalysis of children*. New York: Grove Press.

Klein, M. (1935/1975). A contribution to the psychogenesis of manic-depressive state.
In: *Love, guilty and reparation and other works*. New York: Delta.

Klein, M. and others. (1946/1952). Notes on some schizoid mechanisms.
In: *Developments in psycho-analysis*. London; New York: Karnac.

Petot, J-M. (1979/1991). *Melanie Klein I*. São Paulo: Perspectiva.

Petot, J-M. (1982/1992). *Melanie Klein II*. São Paulo: Perspectiva.

Steiner, J. (1993). *Psychic retreats*. London: Routledge.

Winnicott, D. (1957/1964). Needs of the under-five. In: *The child, the family and the
outside world*. USA: Addison-Wesley Publishing Company.

Winnicott, D. (1958/1990). Psychoanalysis and the sense of guilt. In: *Maturational
processes and the facilitating environment – Studies in the theory of emotional
development*. London: Karnak.

Film reference

City of God. (2002). *Directed by Fernando Meirelles and Kátia Lund*. Screenplay by
Bráulio Mantovani.

6 The schizoid-paranoid and depressive positions

The movement of the mind

*Elisa Maria de Ulhôa Cintra and
Marina F. R. Ribeiro*

The positions are complex and ever-changing configurations, formed by anxieties, defenses, and modes of object relations. The term "position" subtly appears in the 1928 text, *Early Stages of the Oedipus Conflict*, in which Klein presents her theory of mental functioning. This theory, while not denying the libidinal phases proposed by Freud, offers a new perspective of understanding (Baranger, 1981).

The idea of a position immediately evokes the reality of a subject's emotional experience, as they assume a specific stance towards their objects of love and hate. The focus shifts away from the notion of phases or stages that must be passed through along a diachronic line of development and moves closer to the notion of moments and states that alternate synchronously and continuously over time.

According to Klein (1946/1975a, p. 61), the first anxieties are of a persecutory nature: "At the beginning of post-natal life the infant experiences anxiety from internal and external sources. (...) the working of the death instinct within gives rise to the fear of annihilation and that this is the primary cause of persecutory anxiety". Here, the fear for oneself prevails, along with a feeling of being persecuted and threatened. Splitting – between the good and bad objects, between pleasure and displeasure, between inside and outside – is the primary organizing and protective mechanism of mental functioning during the early stages of life.

Such ideas emerged from theories – such as the death drive, which generates anxiety – and from the treatment of many children with severe neurotic disturbances. Rita, who was almost three years old, was one of the cases Klein considered throughout her life. Rita's parents were distraught because, since the birth of her younger brother, the girl had been crying without reason and began to exhibit *terror noturnus*[1] – waking up very frightened, claiming that someone was going to enter her room through the window and attack her genitals. In short, there were many persecutory phantasies that led to an almost total inhibition of play. Additionally, Rita referred to a terrible and threatening mother, while, on the other hand, she reported having another image of a mother, one that was wonderful and protective. From observing

DOI: 10.4324/9781003583035-7

these psychic realities, Klein noted an intense splitting between an excessively bad object and a highly idealized one.

Gratification experiences, on the other hand, stimulate libidinal impulses, love, and the formation of the good object, while frustration experiences stimulate destructive impulses, hatred, and the formation of the bad object. As Rita improved through analysis, a sufficiently good object began to establish itself: neither ideal nor threatening, as was the case initially.

In the face of paranoid-schizoid anxieties, there is fragmentation of the self and objects, resulting from intense splitting. Projection and introjection mechanisms – the breathing of the mind – are also present from the beginning. For Klein, the most primitive form of love is voracious, cannibalistic, and marked by sadism, arrogance, and possessiveness. Primitive love has no regard for the object and is devoid of guilt or responsibility for the other.

What also occurs in the face of persecutory anxieties in the paranoid-schizoid position is the emergence of the fantasy of a perpetually available object, the idealized breast, which provides immediate, unlimited, and permanent gratification. This is a defense mechanism against persecutory anxiety.

In summary, as described in detail in the 1946 paper "Notes on Some Schizoid Mechanisms", the paranoid-schizoid position is characterized by the predominance of splitting, omnipotence, idealization, denial, and omnipotent control over internal and external objects.

In 1935/1975, Klein published the article "A Contribution to the Psychogenesis of Manic-Depressive States", in which she began to think that both child and adult patients enter and exit more depressed or manic states, leading us to understand that psychic constitution itself is of a psychopathological nature; however, with a fluid and transformational character. The title of the article already suggests a fluctuation between different configurations, implying a more dynamic movement and the notion of psychopathological positions that can be transformed and lead to healthier configurations. In the face of the demand to accept losses and enter mourning, patients defended themselves through genuine manic and depressive states. The mourning process and the attempt to free oneself from a primary mode of relationship, which is imprisoning and limiting, only occurred when manic defenses diminished, and some contact with pain and helplessness became possible. Interestingly, the psychoanalyst observed the universality of this process; that is, it was something that occurred in all patients, although in different ways.

Based on the explanatory note drafted by the English Editorial Committee (1996) regarding the 1935 text, we can state that from the first year of life, there is a significant change in the baby's object relations – a shift from relating to a partial object to relating to a total object.

(...) This change brings the ego to a new position in which it is able to identify with its object so that while formerly the infant's anxieties were of a paranoic kind about the preservation of his ego, he now has a more complicated set of ambivalent feelings and depressive anxieties about the condition of his object. He becomes afraid of losing his loved good object, and in addition to persecutory anxieties he experiences guilt for his aggression towards his object and has the urge out of love to repair it. A related change occurs in his defences: he mobilizes manic defences to annihilate persecutors and to deal with his newly experienced guilt and despair. This specific grouping of object relations, anxieties and defences Melanie Klein named the depressive position.

(p. 433)

But what would be the difference between a partial object relation and a total object relation? At the beginning of life, the baby relates to an object that is there to be devoured, consumed, or ignored once it has met its needs. This defines a partial object relation – the love object lacks subject autonomy and is experienced as part or extension of the baby's body. On the other hand, at weaning, the child may begin to glimpse the mother as a total object, a subject with its own rights and desires, and can then start to consider her, driven by love and the fear of losing her. It is the moment when the child becomes more concerned with her preservation and fears her disappearance; the first signs of concern for the other, the ability to care for the other, and feelings of guilt emerge, related to the destructive phantasies that may have occurred prior to this state. The feeling of guilt arises from the debt of love to the object and the fear of losing it. This represents the new position towards the object, which accompanies the identification with the object as another, different from oneself.

Klein (1946/1975, p. 71) had stated: "(...) out of the alternating processes of disintegration and integration develops gradually a more integrated ego, with an increased capacity to deal with persecutory anxiety". The movement of ego integration was always a result of the predominance of the life drive.

On the other hand, in the 1950s, during the analysis of schizophrenic[2] patients, Bion observed in detail the intense psychic movement between the paranoid-schizoid and depressive positions. Within the same session, disintegrated states of the mind were succeeded by integrated states, continuously, in a spiraling circular movement. In these patients, the death drive predominated, leading to the fragmentation of the internal world; therefore, Klein (1940) recognizes the need for the predominance of the loving motion, highlighting the importance of positive experiences with external objects to balance paranoid and depressive anxieties; in particular, the experience with the analyst as a good object can have this effect of organization and cohesion.

The concept of position, unlike the concept of phases, highlighted the dimension of mental functioning complexity, which cyclically integrates and disintegrates in an endless process. In summary, projecting, introjecting, splitting, and ultimately, grieving, integrating, identifying, and repairing are part of a continuous psychic movement. Positions are two ways of experiencing the world and giving meaning to emotional experiences, which succeed and alternate constantly in the human psyche.

Revisiting the ideas presented, we can think of the positions as two different "ways" of reacting to experiences of pleasure and pain, gratification and frustration. These different ways of dealing with experiences are the dynamics of the psychic apparatus, the paranoid-schizoid and depressive dynamics.

In the paranoid-schizoid position, the "law of the jungle" predominates: the love object is someone who is at my service, whom I wish to control and possess, it is a love without consideration. The experience is with partial objects, for example, the breast, a part of the mother – not the mother perceived in her entirety. It is a world of intense and dispersed sensations, in which the anxieties of self-annihilation and persecution predominate.

In the depressive position, on the other hand, the "law of culture" predominates, or respect for the social pact: there is consideration for the love object as someone with rights, understanding and respect for the object's independence, needs, and desires. The experience is with total objects – the mother is perceived as a whole, not as parts. There is the experience of guilt for inflicted aggressions and fear of losing the object, accompanied by an attitude of care and reparation.

Destructive attacks and opportunities for reparation

Let us now elucidate these two ways of experiencing the world, the two positions, through Ravel's opera *L'enfant et les sortilèges*[3] (1920–1924). The opera is one of the first literary materials that Klein (1929) uses to reflect on the creative impulse mobilized by reparative desires after destructive attacks on the object. It appears in the article "Infantile Anxiety-Situations Reflected in a Work of Art and the Creative Impulse", which follows the 1928 article "Early Stages of the Oedipal Conflict".

Still immersed in her investigations into the early Oedipal situation, the sadistic attacks on the object, and the sadism of the archaic superego, Klein (1929) revisits these concepts in her analysis of the opera. We also find in this short text the seed of the concept of positions, implicit in her analysis of the literary material. The description of the events in the opera is an excellent example of the anxieties, defenses, and object relations characteristic of the paranoid-schizoid and depressive positions, which were later postulated in 1935, 1940, 1945/1975, and 1946.

Following Klein's choice of the opera and benefiting from the privilege of knowing her complete works and subsequent developments, we engage here in an exercise to elucidate the predominant anxieties and defenses in the paranoid-schizoid and depressive positions.

The child and the magic spells[4]

The opera *L'enfant et les sortilèges*[5] was composed by Ravel between 1920 and 1924. Written by Colette, the libretto was intended to be a ballet but having just come out of the First World War and dealing with the painful loss of his mother, Ravel became interested in the story and composed a beautiful and extremely sensitive opera. In it, we are brought back to the passion and the intertwining of pleasure and pain that characterize the phantasy life of the child.

The story takes place in a room of an old country house in Normandy, overlooking the garden. It is a calm afternoon; one hears the hiss of a kettle and the purring of a cat. A boy, between six and seven years old, is sitting in front of his homework, visibly bored, in the first scene of the opera. Then a beautiful soprano voice sings: "I don't want to do this homework; I want to go for a walk in the park. I wanted to eat all the cakes in the world, or pull the cat's tail, or cut off the squirrel's tail. I wanted to punish my mother".

The door opens, and the mother enters. All the objects on stage are over-sized to emphasize the boy's smaller size. All we see of the mother is her skirt, apron, and hands – with an affectionate voice, she asks her son if he has done his homework. He then moves defiantly in his chair and sticks out his tongue at her; she walks away and leaves the boy in time-out, with unsweetened tea, locked in the room until dinner.

The boy then has a fit of rage: he throws the teapot and teacup on the floor, starts attacking the squirrel by throwing his pen at it, and forcefully pulls the cat's tail. Using the fireplace tongs, he tries to stir the fire and spills the kettle. The room fills with broken things and steam from the spilled tea. He tears the wallpaper and hangs from the pendulum of an old wall clock, ripping it off. He shouts, "Hooray! No work, no homework. I'm free, bad, and free".

However, the objects the boy mistreated come to life. An armchair refuses to let him sit, but is invited to dance with a sofa, which is also no longer available to him. The armchair, the sofa, and the other chairs unite with the goal of preventing the boy from finding a place to rest, expressing the desire to rid themselves of him forever. The old wall clock, whose pendulum was ripped out, suffers from terrible pain and is unable to keep time; its song is full of pain and despair, and there is a profound distortion in the experience of time. Repeating chaotic and fragmented sounds, it becomes part of the chorus of all the other broken and attacked objects, which are enraged and threaten the cruel boy, who is gradually petrified with fear.

These opening scenes are accompanied by a foxtrot rhythm (the latest trend in the United States in the 1920s), which serves as the backdrop to the dance between the sofa and the little armchair. The furniture, having denied the boy a place to sit and now dancing together, expresses contempt and exclusion, shutting him out of the dance. Another example of exclusion by a loving couple: the teapot, speaking in English, dances with the teacup, which responds in Chinese. These foreign languages only heighten the boy's painful sense of not belonging, of being excluded.

As the sun begins to set, the boy approaches the fireplace seeking warmth. He is then struck by a blazing flame that leaps onto him, singing, "I only warm good boys; the bad ones, I burn!".

The strange, surreal atmosphere intensifies when the shepherds and shepherdesses drawn on the torn wallpaper begin to sing a sorrowful chant: they say they will never be able to meet again, as they have been permanently separated by the boy's sadistic attack. Melancholic, they leave the house in a sorrowful song, in a long farewell procession: yet another intense experience of abandonment.

From the fairy tale that was being read and left unfinished in the torn book, a princess emerges, lamenting her fate in an aria introduced by flutes in a deep tone. In pain, she announces that she must disappear, as the boy's violence has destroyed the world where she lived. He, who just yesterday had fallen in love with the princess, is plunged into desolation and despair as he watches her vanish, evaporating before him.

Searching in vain for the lost page of his book, he sees a small man emerge from the ruins of everything: it is Mr. Arithmetic, or the spirit of mathematics, who makes mistakes and confuses him, speaking incessantly. His clothes are made of numbers, and his hat is shaped like the letter π. He holds a ruler and hops from one side to the other with little dance steps.

Then a beautiful love duet between two cats begins to play, only deepening the boy's sense of exclusion, as it seems that everyone is in love with each other and directs their hatred toward him. Suddenly, the walls of the room disappear, and a bright moonbeam illuminates the scene for the second act.

The garden scene leads the boy, now somewhat dazed, into the frenetic melody of nature: the music of insects, crickets, beetles, the buzzing of bees, the croaking of frogs and toads, the song of nightingales, and the hooting of owls.

Frightened and bewildered, he leans against an old tree that lets out a cry of pain: the boy had played with a knife, injuring its trunk, from which sap was bleeding. Other wounded trees sing and weep in unison, decrying his cruelty.

The dragonfly mourns the loss of its mate, pierced by a needle and pinned to the wall. The bat grieves over the death of the mother of its pups, now dying. This theme has been recurrent since the opera's opening scene – the loss of a mother capable of caring and protecting.

The boy realizes his loneliness and feels out of place; at the center of the scene, objects and animals cry and lament or gather in idyllic pairs. There is a moment of silence, suddenly broken by his desperate cry for his mother. All the animals pounce on the boy, competing for a chance to attack him. In the chaos, a squirrel is injured and rolls over near him. Seeing the animal bleeding in front of him, the boy impulsively forgets his own suffering, takes a scarf from around his neck, and begins to tend to the creature's wounded paw.

Stunned, the animals stop attacking him, back away, and, watching the scene, exclaim: "He took care of the wounded paw that was bleeding". They begin to approach the boy again, recognizing his kindness, and concerned for his injuries, they sing: "He is suffering. He is hurt. He is bleeding. We must close his wound. We don't know how to do it. We need to stop the bleeding.

What to do? He knows how to heal the hurt. We have injured him. A moment ago, he was calling for someone. He shouted a word, 'Mommy'. Someone must hear him there in his nest".

Then, the animals, realizing that the boy's nest was that house in the middle of the garden, begin to guide him back there, singing: "He is good, the boy; he is wise, he is sweet".

The opera concludes with the boy's solo singing "mommy", the magic word that restores harmony on both the psychic and cosmic levels. This corresponds to the recovery of the caring and nurturing mother, reinstating the cosmos where there was chaos[6].

On psychic dynamics

At the beginning of the opera, the boy denies his love and expresses all his hatred and rebellion, along with the desire to dominate and triumph over the entire world. He feels cornered and controlled by an authoritarian mother, who demands an obedience he cannot accept. In his outburst of rage, his omnipotence and desire to need and depend on no one are revealed. This is the moment of manic triumph: he denies any feeling of love and delights in feeling hatred and being bad, for that way, he can be free. He hates having to obey, rebels, screams, and releases his aggression and sadism against all objects. He seeks only immediate pleasure, rejecting work or obedience. He wants to command and exercise sadistic control over objects and animals.

However, when the inanimate objects come to life, they dramatically express their fury and pain from the damage and losses they have suffered. Immersed in a frenetic wave of unconscious action, the boy needs to be shaken by the fury of the animals and objects uniting against him. Then, at the moment he is touched by his own pain and the pain of the wounded squirrel, he manages to come into contact with what he has done. The verbalization of pain and fury makes these feelings even more perceptible and poignant to him.

The little despot becomes humanized and sensitive

At the start of the opera, the boy feels very trapped in that room and with his schoolwork. At that moment, he is also insensitive to the pain and needs of others. He has not yet discovered others as beings separate from himself and acts like a despot: he uses them as mere objects of his pleasure, wanting to dominate them and desiring them to exist solely to serve him. It was necessary for him to go through the experience of being attacked, wounded, and abandoned in order to finally come into contact with his fragility and helplessness. Hearing the wounded squirrel's song of pain and tending to its needs are the events that allow him to recover, within himself, the image of the attentive and loving mother, as he now acts as a protective mother.

The inner world and the turbulent emotions that stir within him begin to color and influence the external world. Thus, at the start of the opera, when he declares that he wants to "eat all the cakes in the world" and "punish the mother", the boy reveals the strength of his voracious oral desires and his impulse to dominate the authority figure, reversing the power dynamic with her. As we've seen, Klein posits that the most primitive form of love is voracious, cannibalistic, and imbued with sadism, arrogance, and possessiveness. The desire to dominate the other, to exert power over them, prevails.

We can assume that the scene of destruction happened on an imaginary plane, within unconscious phantasies. It becomes evident, then, that the "magic spells" or "*sortilèges*" that give the piece its name stem from this magical power of primitive desires and destructiveness, capable of exerting their effects on the world. At first, the magical power is, therefore, only that of breaking and making all sources of security and goodness in the boy's world disappear. The phantasies and acts of destruction have a magical influence on the inanimate world, which becomes, by projection, hostile and attacking; the spell turns against the sorcerer, and all the fury ends up turning back on him.

We can consider that the phantasy life is the sorceress that creates the magical effects (or *sortilèges*) that transformed the world of objects and animals into an "enchanted" world, which falls into disharmony and becomes chaotic. On the other hand, at the end of the opera, the magic word that holds the power to restore cosmic harmony is the invocation of the mother, capable of healing and caring, revealing the other side of the spells or enchantments of the inner world. The act of compassion for the animals' pain and, especially, the care given to the wounded squirrel reveal that the inner scene of phantasy was, at that moment, determined by loving impulses and the recovery of the maternal image, available for care. It is the dominance of this kind of phantasy that creates harmony and unity among the characters.

Oedipus complex and experience of exclusion

There are several moments when the boy feels excluded and abandoned. He is excluded from his mother's approval and company when she punishes him, and later, when he feels that all the objects and animals are leaving him while forming pairs and going off happily, demonstrating their mutual affection.

The experience of exclusion is common in childhood, generating feelings of isolation and of not belonging to the world of adults or other children, which can also occur whenever the mother is absent. The feeling of loneliness is accompanied by the phantasy that the absent mother is gratifying someone else, perhaps the father or another sibling. The child feels enraged at the thought of being excluded from the love between the parents, a theme that repeats itself several times in the opera – the sofa takes the armchair for a dance, and neither is available for the boy; the teapot and teacup speak in a foreign language, and the cats sing their love duet.

On the other hand, other couples were separated by the fury of the little despot and are lamenting their pain, moving the boy: these are the shepherd and the shepherdess, the princess in the book and her knight. This pattern is frequent in childhood phantasies: on the one hand, children want to separate their parents to have each one's absolute love for themselves; on the other, they deeply regret it when such a separation actually happens.

While the child feels the danger of being abandoned by one parent, they can still count on the support of the other. However, when they imagine that both are united against them, they feel utterly helpless. The united parents are greatly feared and transform into persecutors, as they threaten to return all the aggression the child directed at them, leaving no soothing figure to protect them. These are typical anxieties of the Oedipus complex.

It is the control of an authoritarian, bad mother, who frustrates and punishes, and the feeling of being excluded from her love and approval that lead the child to want to punish and attack her. In the opera, the attacks on the house and Mother Nature are symbolic of these desires, revealing the immense ambivalence in the boy's relationship with his mother, marked by both love and hatred. Even before her appearance on stage, at the beginning of the opera, a potentially good and helpful mother had already disappeared from the boy's inner world when he declares that he would like to punish her, anticipating what she might do to him.

Punishment, being left alone, and the mother's expectation that he will reflect on his transgressions, repent for his laziness, and, above all, consider the pain he caused her, turn the mother into a persecutor. At this point, the boy is unable to connect with guilt, repentance, or consideration for her pain; this is still impossible for him. When the mother leaves the room, stating that he is bad, he then tries to lessen the weight of this event through manic defenses, singing "it doesn't matter", "it doesn't matter" (whether she likes me or not), and chanting the words "I don't need anyone". He renounces his capacity for love and proclaims himself "bad", introjecting his mother's accusation. He enters a state of omnipotence and rage, but feels that his inner world is fragmented, in pieces.

The outburst of rage and the projection of his aggression onto the world leave him increasingly weak and impoverished. The discharge of his aggression onto the world of objects and the natural world makes both very threatening, and their retaliatory attack finds the child weakened and without internal resources to defend himself. One example of vengeful attacks is that of "Mr. Arithmetic", who moves incessantly and intrusively to disturb and confuse the boy. At this point in the opera, the *staccato*[7] of the music can be heard, indicating the state of fragmentation and disorder of his inner world.

In the second act, the scene shifts from inside the house to the garden, and the persecutory atmosphere eases, being replaced by the pain and lamentation of the wounded trees and the animals mourning their lost loved ones. The atmosphere is one of mourning, and both the child and the listener are called to observe the characteristics of the creatures, their beauty, and the love they feel for each other.

All these elements deepen the sense of sorrow and prepare the boy for contact with his own pain. He can then confront two realities: from his point of view, the natural world had been the object of his domination and sadism, serving to test his strength and power; but from the animals' point of view, he was the unwanted invader who destroyed life and attacked what was most dear to them. The fairy tale princess speaks of the dismantling of the world she inhabited, and the shepherds who formed happy pairs on the wallpaper are brutally separated: the fabric of their world was torn. Listening to the lament and accounts of all, the boy began to realize the effects of his aggression.

It is also interesting to compare the animals' accusations to those of the mother. Although the former repeatedly accuse the boy, much like the mother had done at the beginning of the opera, the sorrowful, loving appeal and the sad tone they impart, lamenting the catastrophe caused by sadism, create the conditions for the boy to enter into a new reflection on the events, enabling him to recognize his guilt; whereas the mother's accusations left him impervious to it. At that earlier moment, he had not yet fully experienced his own helplessness, and the mother's authoritarian tone prevented him from hearing her. In the end, the boy realizes that the animals are mourning their dead and grieving for all that has been lost and destroyed. The pain he feels, along with the animals' pain, and the feelings of guilt and longing for the lost harmony help him step away from the grandiose, all-powerful feeling and move toward recognizing his helplessness and needs, forcing him to confront the painful feelings of guilt over the irreparable losses and damage.

The small gesture of reparation through caring for the squirrel's paw is recognized and amplified by the animals that gather to help and bring it to the mother. This gesture may be a representation of the movement toward integrating his shattered internal world, something that begins to occur when he invokes the mother, thus rescuing the imago of a good, loving person capable of caring. Only after invoking her – which is nothing but another name for his own capacity to love – does he become able to notice the injured squirrel and care for it. Let us recall that, before addressing the good mother, the boy had been profoundly moved by the pain and lament of the wounded animals. He had felt the pain of being attacked and injured and experienced the remorse of having inflicted attacks; subsequently, he wished to repair them.

Aggressiveness leads to the fragmentation of the internal world, and there must be a predominance of loving motion for integration to occur. This latter is the condition of possibility for one to admire the beauty of nature and to have an aesthetic experience of the world. When the scene shifts from the house to the garden, the music, initially agitated and frantic, begins to calm with the painful laments of mourning and sorrow. There are many references to the beauty of nature's forms: loving it is only possible when a more depressive dynamic is reached, and the desire to care can be recovered. Thinking and feeling involve a certain sadness…

At first, the mother wants her son to conform to her expectations and gives him little space to develop his own interest in learning. He feels confined within the closed room and his mother's designs. When he gives free rein to his fury, a more expanded scene emerges, where objects and animals gain voices and lives that give new meanings to what he is experiencing. If he was furious, feeling humiliated and abandoned by his mother, her anger caused everything to be perceived as chaotic and turned against him. This is a fantastic projection of his own rage and the mother's negative feelings directed against the child.

Phantasized attacks on the inside of the maternal body

The trees in the garden complained of having been injured by the boy. Melanie Klein thought that harming the object might be linked to the desire to enter it, to see what is inside, to know how it came into existence; ultimately, to an epistemophilic drive. But, having injured the object, he realizes he cannot uncover the mystery of his own existence. The desire to harm and dominate objects is also the desire to know them internally, in their true essence. This speculative curiosity, which seeks to manipulate, is also a sign of possessiveness, the desire to dominate and control the other in their enigmatic capacity to appear and disappear on their own, as happens with primary objects.

In this boy, there is the need to "enter the tree": a combination of the desire for a fusion-like, deep love, the desire to belong to the same space as the other, as in gestation, with a sadistic element that seeks to invade the mother's interior to take out everything good that might be denied to him and given to another. This, then, is the voracious dimension of love. The desire to dominate by force can transform into the desire to dominate through the act of knowing. We can say that every desire to understand contains a sadistic element, a desire to capture and imprison the other and its enigma. For the desire to know to be freed from this tendency to imprison the other, it is necessary to respect their autonomy and freedom, a theme addressed in the opera in the melodious lament of the squirrel, trapped in a cage.

Let us return to the dialogue between the boy and the squirrel, after the latter was freed from the cage where it had been imprisoned. The animal sings a poignant song and expresses the pain of being confined and deprived of freedom. The boy tries to justify having caged it, but hearing his interlocutor poetically express his feeling of pain awakens empathy in the boy, who had also been trapped and confined. This awakens in him the awareness of his internal world, the perception that he exists separately from others; and through his own pain, thus objectified in the squirrel's song, he becomes aware of the value of freedom.

The relationship with the squirrel and its need to be free marks the shift from a mode of relating to the other through domination to a relationship of admiration and desire to know. In other words, the desire to possess, control, and dominate is replaced by the desire to know. It is necessary to respect the other's freedom in order to desire them in this new way, as an other.

Being trapped in the room may represent the boy's feeling of loneliness and isolation. He needed the mother to help him glimpse something of his internal world, but this remained as a closed and inaccessible dimension, bringing a feeling of exclusion. He needed the mother to recognize him in his passion, that is, both in his power of destructiveness and in his capacity to love. While the mother demanded blind obedience to the established rules, the boy became rebellious, until the wounded animals and the experience of his own fury and pain led him to a deeper connection with his imaginary world, and he could enter the depressive position.

The character journeys in this opera from learning *about* something to the experience of learning *from* his own emotional experience, transitioning through the anxieties and defenses of the schizoid-paranoid and depressive positions; in this way, the little despot, who we all are, becomes humanized.

Notes

1 TN: Free translation: night terrors.
2 In the 1950s, maintaining the classical analytic framework in these cases was considered impossible by some psychoanalysts, making it something innovative and supported by the Kleinian group.
3 TN: The Child and the Magic Spells.
4 TN: All quotations from the opera The Child and the Spells were provided by the translator.
5 Sortilèges are magic spells. One could think that magic spells arise from the imagination and that the power of imagination permeates the world, coloring it in more hostile or more friendly tones.
6 In an understanding of the importance of survival, within the inner world, of the figure of the nurturing mother, Clarice Lispector writes: "mother is not dying".
7 TN: In opera, staccato refers to a style of singing or playing where the notes are performed in a short, detached manner, creating a crisp and distinct sound. This technique involves articulating each note separately rather than connecting them smoothly, which can add a sense of urgency or playfulness to the music.

References

Baranger, W. (1981). *Posição e objeto na obra de Melanie Klein*. Translation: Maria Nestrovsky Folberg. Porto Alegre: Artes Médicas.

Klein, M. (1928/1986). Early stages of the Oedipus conflict. In: *The selected Melanie Klein*. New York: The Free Press.

Klein, M. (1929/1948). Infantile anxiety-situations reflected in a work of art and the creative impulse. In: *Contributions to psycho-analysis*. London: The Hogarth Press.

Klein, M. (1935/1975). A contribution to the psychogenesis of manic-depressive states. In: *Love, guilt and reparation other works*. New York: Dell Publishing Co.

Klein, M. (1940/1975). Mourning and it relation to manic-depressive states. In: *Love, guilt and reparation and other works*. New York: Dell Publishing Co.

Klein, M. (1945/1975). The Oedipus complex in the light of early anxieties. In: *Love, guilt and reparation other works*. New York: Dell Publishing Co.

Klein, M. (1946/1975a). Some theoretical conclusions regarding the emotional life of the infant. In: *Envy and gratitude and other works*. New York: The Free Press.

Klein, M. (1946/1975b). Notes on some schizoid mechanism. In: *Envy and gratitude and other works*. New York: The Free Press.

Ravel, M. (1925) L'enfant et les sortilèges: Fantaisie lyrique en deux parties. https://youtu.be/MFViB9vrB1E?si=qonhxmT_X-mYCddp. Accessed in: 10/01/2024.

7[1] The feminine position

A theory on femininity and masculinity[2]

Marina F. R. Ribeiro

First, we would like to revisit the concepts of position and phase, explained in the chapter on paranoid-schizoid and depressive positions. In 1932[3], Klein used both expressions: phase of femininity and feminine position, making no distinction between them. However, phase conveys something transient, suggesting a transition to another level, another phase; in other words, it inherently carries the idea of development, of overcoming. Position, on the other hand, is a place occupied in response to an emotional experience, referring to the idea of interchangeable, mutable states, of various psychic organizations in response to experience. Based on this understanding, we believe that the concept of position brings forth the idea of a psychic dynamism more aligned with emotional experiences, leading to a better understanding of the complexity of Klein's theory today[4].

According to Herrmann and Alves Lima (1982, p. 17), it was necessary for a woman to dedicate herself to understanding the female experience in order for the Freudian view of equating the masculine Oedipal trajectory with the feminine one, prevalent in psychoanalysis during the 1920s, to be modified, and for the specificities of the feminine to be considered. Indeed, in addition to bringing new understandings of anxieties specific to girls, Klein (1932) refers to the feminine position as an experience shared by both sexes, something that had not yet been expressed in psychoanalysis until then.

The psychoanalyst then invites us to observe the initial experience of life, predominantly bodily, synthesized in the breast–mouth image. The baby's first reality is the maternal unconscious; the idea of a system of communicating vessels is intriguing: "The baby begins to be and is in relation to the mother, with the maternal body, with the breast that nourishes and comforts it[5]". The mother experiences this deeply, identifying with the baby, lending her thoughts and cultural heritage to the child, in a system of communicating vessels... (Herrmann and Alves Lima, 1982, p. 17).

Klein (1932) postulates that the main feminine anxiety concerns internal damage, the fear of having her interior attacked and destroyed; for the author, castration anxiety in girls is secondary. From this perspective, object relations are present from the very beginning, with their intense ambiguities, love

DOI: 10.4324/9781003583035-8

and hate. The girl, in her phantasy, imagines attacks on the interior of the maternal body and its contents, possible babies. The receptive characteristic of the female sexual organ comes to the fore; in other words, the different bodily experience between boys and girls becomes a subject of reflection in Klein's texts.

It is important to consider that Freud (1926) questioned castration in girls, highlighting the difficulty of understanding castration anxiety when it has already occurred. And, right at the beginning of the text "Female Sexuality", he writes: "We have, after all, long given up any expectation of a neat parallelism between male and female sexual development" (Freud, 1931/2024, p. 227).

We can think that Klein followed the "clues" left by Freud. At the end of the 1932 text, she briefly contrasts some Freudian ideas regarding the Oedipal trajectory of girls. Like Freud (1931/2024), she understands that the girl's attachment to her father is deeply affected by her initial attachment to her mother, and that one is built upon the other, resulting in the fact that, in adulthood, women's relationships with their husbands tend to repeat their conflicts with their mothers.

However, in a different way, Freud's conception held that the girl's exclusive attachment to her mother would last until the age of five. Nevertheless, Klein (1932) highlights the early presence of the father, first encountered as an internal object in the mother's mind.

The mother – the maternal body, the breast, the maternal unconscious – is the primary object, the first object of identification for babies of both sexes. This observation, likely drawn from Klein's personal experience with motherhood and also based on her work with very young children, was fundamental to a perspective of understanding different from the Freudian one – according to which the "discovery" of the vagina would only occur in adult life.

Klein (1932 and 1945) follows a different direction. A woman does indeed have psychic representations of her own sex: early vaginal sensations, the potential to bear children, and, later, the breasts.

In this regard, Chasseguet-Smirgel (1988, p. 31) warns:

How can we truly suppose that the girl is unaware of possessing a vagina, when Freud attributes to dreams, in the "Metapsychological Supplement to the Theory of Dreams" (1915), the ability to perceive early on all organic modifications? Why would the unconscious' powers to know what is happening within our bodily intimacy not extend to the vagina? How could there not be, for the boy, a foreknowledge of a complementary organ to his own, when Freud, on the other hand, postulates the existence of innate phantasies?[6]

It is common for anyone observing children at play to witness the scene of two children between the ages of two and three discovering their bodily differences. This curiosity – what Klein (1928) named the epistemophilic drive – is linked to primordial questions, the great enigmas of existence: Where did I come from? Who am I? What is my body like? What are the bodies of adult caregivers like? What is the relationship between them, etc.? The dyads are thus experienced by the baby and always summoned and present in the infantile part of the adult: breast–mouth; vagina–penis, inside and outside, self–other, presence–absence.

From these primordial experiences, Klein (1932) postulates the concept of the feminine position, which consists of the infant's initial and early identification with the mother. Around six months, the infant turns toward the father, identified with the mother. At this moment, there is a first glimpse that the mother is an "other" and that the father is the mother's other. For Klein, the penis (partial object/paranoid-schizoid position) is first found within the mother. In other words, the father is found in the mother's gaze, in the maternal unconscious, the baby's first reality. Thus, in contrast to Freud, she understands that the father is present from the beginning in the mother's mind; that is, the breast contains the penis.

With the goal of reflecting on issues related to sexual identity, in her 1945 text, Klein articulates the concepts of the feminine position, the depressive position, and the early Oedipus complex, but not with the paranoid-schizoid position, which was conceptualized a year later, in 1946. With the concept of the depressive position, she revisits libidinal positions and, therefore, the feminine position – a position we believe is connected to an interesting theoretical construction of femininity and masculinity, but which did not gain further development within Klein's theory.

The feminine position is the foundational experiential support for the later psychic constructions of masculinity and femininity to emerge. We understand that the formation of sexual identity is composed of a complex blend of masculine and feminine identifications, which do not necessarily align with biological sex. There is great plasticity in psychic constitution, but it always arises from early object relations and the libidinal charge that permeates these relations.

Articulating the two concepts – feminine position and depressive position – can lead us to interesting reflections; for if we are always within the realm of a constant and continuous process of construction and articulation between a subject and an object, in which alterity is always uncertain and depressive, femininity and masculinity dialogue with these issues. For identification to occur, a depressive delineation of self–other must happen. We therefore emphasize that the feminine position is a beginning of self–other differentiation, and also a beginning of the differentiation between breast and penis, mother and father, or between the adult caregivers who perform maternal and paternal functions, regardless of biological sex designation.

Both girls and boys identify with maternal/feminine attributes and turn toward the father, identified with the mother's femininity. For male infants, in the feminine position, what is at stake is the possibility of sublimating their feminine components. Successfully navigating this phase allows, in adulthood, for a man to appreciate feminine attributes without needing to denigrate them (Klein, 1932).

A possible attitude of male depreciation toward women can be understood as a defensive movement in relation to a mother/woman who has become threatening in the psyche of the male infant. This occurs when feelings of envy and hatred toward the mother predominate. Conversely, when loving feelings predominate – that is, more depressive and reparative feelings – contact with the feminine and its interiority seems to endow men with surprising psychic qualities, among them, the ability to appreciate a woman's femininity.

For girls, this identification with the mother in the phase of femininity exerts a pull toward the archaic. At each phase (menarche, defloration, first pregnancy, and menopause), the girl (and later the woman) is drawn back to identification with the mother.

Kristeva (1999) emphasizes that it was Klein who proposed the "first psychoanalytic model of sexuation founded on the couple[7]". The combined or coupled parents are the archaic reference of the parental couple, both in the baby's mind and in the mother's unconscious.

On this subject, Klein (1945/1996, p. 419) writes: "The sexual development of the child is inextricably bound up with his object relations and with all the emotions which from the beginning mould his attitude to mother and father".

The feminine position for infants of both sexes would be this archaic reservoir of unconscious phantasy, shared with the mother's body/psyche, with mutual affectation between the baby and the mother through the unconscious phantasy of the pair: mother–female baby and mother–male baby. The metaphor of the communicating vessels, mentioned earlier, expresses this mutual affectation, marked by corporeality.

Femininity, in its sense of passivity, receptivity, and interiority, is not exclusive to women. Men share and compose their masculinity from this maternal and feminine universe, albeit in a different way.

Given that our origins are feminine (André, 1995), the primary object is feminine, marking the trajectory of infants of both sexes, with subtle differences. Klein realized this in the late 1930s, a bold thought for psychoanalytic knowledge at the time.

The concept of the feminine position also had significant developments in the theoretical constructions of Florence Guignard, an author we will now introduce, highlighting her contributions regarding the formation of femininity in women.

The primary maternal and primary feminine: a brief presentation of Florence Guignard's thought

Florence Guignard (1997, 2000, and 2002), a contemporary French psychoanalyst, proposes the distinction between two psychic spaces in which the configurations of initial identifications with the mother are organized.

Guignard (2000) considers the hypothesis of the existence of two stages of the feminine, in which the initial identifications with the primary object are organized. The first stage is that of the primary maternal (between two and three months of life); the second is that of the primary feminine (around six months).

The space of the primary maternal constitutes the internal space of the instinctual investments of the first identificatory relationships with the mother, violently imprinting the unknown of the object onto the child's psyche-soma and directing the drives toward the object[8]. Inspired by Laplanche's theory (1988), Guignard (2000) characterizes the unknown of the object as the "enigmatic".

The space of the primary feminine is where what Klein termed the femininity phase or feminine position is established. The child identifies with the mother's desire for the father – it is an identification with the desire of the other (mother) for the other (father). This occurs at the threshold of the depressive position, at the end of the omnipotent and narcissistic mother–baby dyad, and in the face of the first Oedipal triangulation – the early Oedipus, as named by Klein (1928). It is the moment of deidealization: the baby is not everything to the mother – she desires another, the father, the third or his representative. Guignard (2002) notes that, at this moment, the daughter must identify with the one who deprived her of her omnipotent status as the mother's sole object of love: the sexual mother.

> I consider the "primary feminine" to be the psychic space that develops in relation to the first observable triangulation in the human being. It is the initial place of the desire for the Other-of-the-Other, of absence, negativity, mutual abandonment, and, consequently, of the entire potential for mourning processes. The proper establishment of this space will determine the economic balance of psychic bisexuality in relation to the individual's biological sex.
>
> (Guignard, 2000, p. 140)[9]

From the organization of the psychic space of the primary feminine, there is an increase in introjective identifications. A more defined inside and outside, a self, an other, and an other of the other begin to form. Like Klein, Guignard (2000) considers that the core of the ego is constituted by introjective identifications, and since these are initially feminine, the fate of the ego becomes linked to the fate of the feminine.

In 1945, Klein writes that the first object introjected is the mother's breast, a breast that contains the penis; that is, the image of the combined parents, the archaic reference of the parental couple.

Introjective identifications of the primary maternal and primary feminine are necessary for the economic balance of psychic bisexuality, both for boys and girls. However, due to the destiny of becoming a woman and a mother, these identifications will be even more demanded in relation to the bodily ego of the girl. Guignard's (2002) hypothesis is that the investment in the maternal and feminine by an adult woman and mother functions as a seesaw, as figure and ground, and under the sign of guilt.

To summarize, the space of the primary maternal constitutes the internal space of the instinctual investments of the first identificatory relationships with the mother, violently imprinting the unknown of the object onto the child's psyche-soma and directing the drives toward the object.

The space of the primary feminine is where what Klein called the feminine position is established. The child identifies with the mother's desire for the father; it is an identification with the desire of the other (mother) for the other (father). This happens at the threshold of the depressive position, at the end of the omnipotent and narcissistic mother–baby dyad, and in the face of the first Oedipal triangulation – the early Oedipus, as Klein named it in 1928.

Finally, let us give voice to the poet Mia Couto (1990), who is able to express the experience incomparably well in *Woman of Me* – the feminine is, then, the woman of me, or, we might say, the feminine in me:

> That night, the hours ran all round me, like sleepless clockhands. All I wanted was to forget me.

> (…) In this while, she came in. She was a woman whose soft eyes cast a moist film upon the room. She wandered around, as if she did not believe in her own presence. Her fingers travelled over the furniture in distracted affection. Who knows, perhaps she was walking in her slumber, maybe that reality held more in the way of fiction for her? I wanted to warn her that she was mistaken, that that was not her correct address.

> (…) But this unknown woman was provoking me with the descent of her cleavage. …, But thanks to the intruder's arts, I was disappearing, intermittent, from existence. I was unfulfilling myself. And when I appealed to myself to return to reason, I could not even get as far as that austere judge, my brain. All because of the woman's voice: it recalled the gentle murmur of a spring, the seduction of a return to times beyond, when there was no before.

> (…) (…) What did she come to do, then? For the more she took possession, the more I grew uneasy. The envoy continued:

> — Don't you understand? I have come to find a place within you. She explained her reasons: only she kept the eternal gestation of the sources. Without being her, I remained incomplete, made whole only in the arrogance of halves. In her, I found not a woman who belonged to me but the woman of me, the one who, from now on, would ignite me with each moon.
> — Let me be born in you. (Mia Couto, 2017, p. 127–133)[10] [11]

If identifications are what remains of passions – what remains after everything has been forgotten – our primary identifications are feminine. The feminine – common to both sexes – is understood as the term that designates the first position, the matrix of origins, the primordial encounter with the mother, the experience of an absence of representation. In other words, the unrepresentable, the realm of the archaic, of primal repression.

It is surprising that Melanie Klein wrote about the feminine position as early as 1928 and 1932.

Notes

1 TN: Translation done by Eduardo Jefferson de Oliveira, cmo.edu@gmail.com.
2 Some of the contents of this chapter are also present in the book *From Mother into Daughter: The Transmission of Femininity* (Ribeiro, 2011).
3 Specifically in the texts: "The Effects of Early Archaic Anxiety Situations on the Sexual development of the Girl" and "The Effects of Early Archaic Anxiety Situations on the Sexual Development of the Boy".
4 We can consider that the feminine position is in a transitional area between the paranoid-schizoid and depressive positions, sharing anxieties and defenses from these two states of mind.
5 TN: Translation provided by the translator.
6 TN: Free translation done by the translator.
7 TN: Free translation done by the translator.
8 It becomes clear that Guignard links Freud's theory of drives with Klein's theory of object relations.
9 TN: The quotation was translated by the translator.
10 Only a few sentences from the story are quoted.
11 TN: Free translation done by the translator.

References

André, J. (1995). *Aux origines féminines de la sexualitá*. Paris: Presses Universitaires de France. (Translation: On the Feminine Origins of Sexuality).

Chasseguet-Smirgel. (1988). *As duas árvores do jardim – ensaios psicanalíticos sobre o papel do pai e da mãe no psiquismo*. Porto Alegre: Imago. (Translation: The two trees in the garden – Psychoanalytic essays about the role of the father and the mother in the psyche).

Couto, M. (1990). Woman of me. In: *Every mand is a race*. Translated by David Brookshaw. Johannesburg: Heinemann Pulishers.

Freud, S. (1926/1959). *Inhibitions, symptoms and anxiety*. New York; London: W. W. Norton and Company. Translated by Alix Strachey, revised and edited by James Strachey.

Freud, S. (1931/2024). Female sexuality. In: *The revised standard edition of the complete psychological works of Sigmund Freud*. Maryland: Rowman & Littlefield. Translation by Joan Riviere and edited by Ernest Jones.

Guignard, F. (1997). *O infantil ao vivo. Reflexões sobre a situação analítica*. (Tradução: Marilda Pedreira). Rio de Janeiro: Imago. (Translation: The infantile in the live: reflections on the analytic situation).

Guignard, F. (2000). *Cartas ao objeto*. (Tradução: Marilda Pedreira). Rio de Janeiro: Imago. (Translation: Letters to the object).

Guignard, F. (2002). *La relacion mère-fille. Entre partage et clivage. Collection de la SEPEA*. Paris: In Press Éditions. (Translation: The mother-daughter relationship: between sharing and splitting. SEPEA Collection).

Herrmann, F., & Alves Lima, A. (1982). *Melanie Klein – Coleção Grandes Cientistas Sociais*. (Coordenador: Florestan Fernandes). São Paulo: Ática. (Translation: Melanie Klein – Great Social Scientists Collection).

Klein, M. (1928/1986). *Early stages of the Oedipus conflict. In: The selected Melanie Klein*. New York: The Free Press.

Klein, M. (1932/1960). The effects of early anxiety-situations on the sexual development of the girl. In: *The psychoanalysis of children*. New York: Grove Press.

Klein, M. (1945/1975). The Oedipus complex in the light of early anxieties. In: *Love, guilt and reparation other works*. New York: Dell Publishing Co.

Klein, M. (1946/1975). Notes on some schizoid mechanism. In: *Envy and gratitude and other works*. New York: The Free Press.

Kristeva, J. (1999). *Le génie féminin: la vie, la folie, les mots: Hannah Arendt, Melanie Klein, Colette*. Paris: Fayard. (Translation: The Feminine Genius: Life, Madness, Words: Hannah Arendt, Melanie Klein, Colette).

Laplanche, J. (1988). *Teoria da sedução generalizada e outros ensaios*. (Tradução: Doris Vasconcellos). Porto Alegre: Artes Médicas. (Translation: Theory of generalized seduction and other essays).

8 Envy and gratitude

Some notes

*Elisa Maria de Ulhôa Cintra and
Marina F. R. Ribeiro*

As we saw earlier, Melanie Klein (1957/1975) published the text *Envy and Gratitude* in the 1950s. In it, she highlighted the manifestation of destructive impulses that take the form of envy, corresponding to the desire to attack and destroy the good object, which is the foundation of psychic health. In this chapter, we will delve deeper into this theme.

The object par excellence of envy is the life-giving object: creativity, fertility, generosity, and plenitude. In other words, envy targets those attributes that the young child ascribes to the maternal figure and, later, to the paternal figure. It is difficult to accept the beauty, radiance, and presence of the mother and caregivers – those who are providers or possessors of knowledge, gifts, or other goods one wishes to have.

The tragedy of envy is that, by directing its destructiveness toward what could be attained, it prevents the assimilation of the good object and the processes of psychic integration. When envy is absent, the introjection of the good object – complete and intact – creates a nucleus that generates life drives. If this introjection fails, the rest of development is compromised. The rooting of the good object in the ego is the only means of preventing the destructive power of envy.

For Klein (1957), envy has a constitutional basis – an idea worth examining, as it was one of the aspects of her theory that was poorly understood. We understand that our author did not believe in a genetic component. She observed that some newborns were more capable of using the good object than others, showing themselves more resolved in relation to their satisfaction, with greater tolerance for frustration and a greater capacity to experience gratitude. They would thus be better equipped to benefit from what the environment has to offer.

But what does it mean to be better equipped? It means being less greedy, as greed makes gratification difficult – intense sucking constricts the capillaries, and the flow of milk is reduced. An intolerance for frustration leads to hatred and the desire to attack and destroy the frustrating object. Greater greed always gives the impression of being unsatisfied, which fuels envy in a destructive, self-reinforcing cycle, hindering development.

DOI: 10.4324/9781003583035-9

How can we understand that there is a potential for the experience of envy from the very beginning of life? One possibility is to consider that the experience of birth, by promoting the exit from intrauterine homeostasis, produces a loss of pleasure and a comparison between the current situation and the memory of that lost plenitude. This simple difference, which is the human existential condition, gives rise to a voracious desire to recover what was lost. Voracious desire for something unattainable is fertile ground for envy.

We think that instead of using the term "constitutional", Melanie Klein should have used the term "structural". If we compare the intrauterine situation with the baby's state after birth, we see that the plenitude and sense of undivided being are different in both moments. No mother will be able to create a sense of unity comparable to prenatal unity – this situation creates an insurmountable pleasure differential. Thus, envy is destined to happen, as it is nothing more than the effect of comparison between prenatal plenitude and ecstasy and the relatively painful and uncomfortable situation of post-natal life.

Moreover, birth provokes persecutory anxieties, and to combat them, phantasy creates an idealized object corresponding to the fullness of intra-uterine life, a sort of model or paradigm of absolute satisfaction. The need to idealize, derived from the universal longing for a state of plenitude, whether prenatal or stemming from the experience of satisfaction, gives rise to the desire to be free of all pain and persecutory anxiety (Klein, 1957/1975).

There is a libidinal component to envy, a nostalgia for a state of full satisfaction once experienced and lost, mingled with hatred, resentment, and the feeling that something has become forever unattainable. If the real breast does not provide that level of pleasure offered by the ideal breast, there arises the feeling of being wronged and the desire to destroy the real breast. Considering, then, that the real breast can never match the imaginary fullness of intrauterine life, there will always be space for envy to emerge. The same can be said of romantic encounters at any level, as there is always a gap between what is desired and what is achieved.

For this reason, we state that envy can be considered constitutional; that is, it arises from the discontinuity between two different experiences of pleasure, in whose imaginary elaboration greed emerges. This is the original structure of human desire: insatiable. And this makes envy exist as a consequence of this voracious structure – we simply want everything! And reality, even when it is quite generous, never manages to satisfy everything.

In fact, we can say that envy is part of the structure of human desire, highlighting its insatiable aspect. The excessive nature of the drive life is the "deadly" trait. The more "benign" aspect (of this "deadly" trait) is wanting more, which could coexist with frustration and transform. The more "malignant" aspect is wanting to destroy and annihilate the object that frustrates and separate from it, denying dependence.

Although envy is the prototypical expression of the death drive and its power of dissolution, it is addressed to Eros – it is the force directed at undoing the original knot between the life and death drives, with its objective being to perform a silent and sinister work of dissolving erotic bonds, in order to destroy dependence on the sources of life, pleasure, and plenitude.

What is most intolerable is the unconscious phantasy that the idealized object has so much and gives nothing. This is what makes the reflection on envy so interesting, the fact that, being the ultimate manifestation of the death drive, it arises from the very core of the life drive, from the intensity of desire. It is envy that seeks to break the ties with the love object, with the aim of destroying Eros, to free oneself from all dependence, and in doing so also annihilates the capacity for association, which is necessary for thinking. Envy prevents the formation of associative bonds necessary for the construction of thinking – it is an attack on linking (Bion, 1959/1988). When there is tolerance for pain and frustration, it signals that one can wait longer for satisfaction, that one can keep alive the memory of satisfaction and a state of gratitude: thinking itself can emerge in the presence of tolerated frustration, when there is hope that satisfaction will return, for it is this very tolerance for the pain of absence and this hope that make thinking possible, enabling the necessary associative connections.

Envy is always directed at the good breast, which is the prototype of maternal goodness, inexhaustible patience and generosity, affection, compassion, and understanding. The good object is the foundation of hope and trust. But the object is only good if there is the capacity to "receive", to embrace its "goodness".

The mother has the ability to create an atmosphere of trust and care – the flow of milk, the presence that offers companionship, touch, stimulation, playfulness, facial expressions, listening, nourishment, attention, putting some experiences into words, narration, teaching how to contain and overcome impasses; in short, all the work of erotic connection that leads to love, intelligence, meaningful activities, and the pleasure of playing and thinking.

According to our author, the impermanence of the object and its inability to meet the insatiability of desire give rise to hatred and resentment, which are encompassed under the name "envy". Envy arises because there is an oscillation, sometimes unbearable, between having and losing this world of maternal gifts – and perceiving oneself as too dependent. There is an oscillation between the lack and the excess of stimuli resulting from greed, frustration, and the affects mobilized by the situation.

Jealousy stems from envy, for behind the aspiration to the exclusive possession of the love object that characterizes it lies the hatred of having to depend on it, the envy of what it can offer, and the desire to exert control over it. We can distinguish the following nuances: greed is the craving to suck everything, leaving it dry; envy is the desire to spoil the object, to deposit malice, excrement, and bad parts inside the mother in order to destroy her, but especially to destroy her creativity. Envying is an attack on desire and desiring, with its procession of torments, and it involves attempting to diminish the value of the object, demeaning it until it becomes less desirable.

Fully enjoying generates gratitude, a feeling that diminishes envy and greed. Gratitude is the foundation of the ability to appreciate and savor the good moments and qualities offered to us. The sum of happy experiences with the good breast allows for the good introjection of this object, which functions as a nucleus of love and protection and will forever be the ultimate source of the subject's life drive. Gratitude deepens the ability to "use the good breast", and the better the breast becomes, the more gratitude there is: "through processes of projection and introjection, through inner wealth given out and re-introjected, an enrichment arid deepening of the ego comes about" (Klein, 1957/1975, p. 189). Gratitude is intimately linked to generosity.

This is the core of all ethical values of the subject. It is the foundation of the subject's trust in the world and their "trustworthiness" – that is, their ability to commit to values and practices, and to maintain that commitment over time. Contact with this internal reservoir of trustworthiness forms the basis for the ability to tolerate frustrations, which allows for the experience of gratitude. Furthermore, the firm introjection of the good object protects against character alterations that stem from oral and anal traits – excessive ambition, rivalry, desire for control, and possessiveness. Even the most voracious tendencies of infantile sexuality can be integrated into the ego, enriching it; problems arise when this integration is not possible.

Klein (1957/1975) states that those who have not firmly established the good internal object, when feeling threatened and persecuted, lose complete contact with this internal reservoir of trustworthiness and are driven to act recklessly, as they believe they have nothing to lose. Various degrees of disturbances are possible, including character alterations that lead to acting out and transgressing laws of various kinds; on the other hand, losing contact with this internal reservoir of security leads to acute states of anxiety and helplessness, such as in panic syndrome, autistic retreats, and contact inhibitions and phobias.

Our author differentiates structuring splits from fragmenting splits. Envy arises precisely from the inability to preserve the good object from attacks, which would form a good egoic foundation. Pathogenic splits are those that create extremely good and bad objects, as these cannot be assimilated by the ego and thus do not nourish it. Highly idealized models remain dissociated – they are internal voices that orbit the ego but do not become part of it, and the person cannot act or think independently, remaining subjected to commands, injunctions from these phantasmal others. The idealizations of the object do not hold up and collapse, creating the need to constantly change the object of love.

Indeed, one way of avoiding the work of processing hostility and envy toward the primary object is to find new loves that can be idealized and admired, thus magically bypassing the need to deal with negative emotions. Negative emotions that arise simultaneously with positive emotions create an intolerable conflict. Therefore, one seeks new loves toward which only positive emotions seem to exist.

When it has not been possible to sufficiently enjoy the maternal breast, the first phantasies of jealousy emerge. In such cases, paranoid and schizoid mechanisms predominate, and neither envy nor jealousy can be relieved. However, when these mechanisms give way to the depressive position, the child accepts the loss of the absolute possession of the mother, making it easier to share her with others.

The absolute feeling of exclusion and abandonment is at the root of the "combined parent figure" – a typical phantasy of the early Oedipal complex, linked to archaic affects of jealousy and envy. It is an extreme figuration of the "excluded third" in other words, the mother gratifies the father in every way that love can imagine, forming a combined figure with him and making a power alliance against the child, who bitterly feels their abandonment and helplessness.

The envy experienced in the primary relationship with the mother gives rise to other forms of envy, such as penis envy, mentioned by Freud. Melanie Klein discerns the logic governing all forms of envy. The envious person seeks self-sufficiency and rejects dependency – they want to possess the source of all their pleasures and will envy the breast and the penis, which are metaphors for everything that can be desired: the capacity to offer pleasure, give life, provide nourishment, energy, love, money, talent, or understanding. Thus, the equation breast–penis is formed, as both organs symbolize life, potency, creativity – objects par excellence of envy.

The defenses against envy are omnipotence, denial, and splitting, as well as idealization and denigration. There are two contradictory ways to defend against envy: either through extreme devaluation or through excessive exaltation of the object and its gifts – these are tendencies to create gods and demons. Extreme division occurs when it is not possible to discriminate and integrate relative forms of love and hate.

Exalted forms of splitting the object – in passion, for instance – are considered delusional. Reality constantly demonstrates that pure forms of absolute good or evil exist only in the imagination; thus, the ideal object quickly becomes a persecutor, as it is the source of excessively high demands. Every idealization harbors within itself a denied envy and unneutralized destructiveness, which is ready to explode in the form of hatred and the desire to destroy. Extreme affects do not stabilize, and hatred does not transform into love. The dynamic of the very good and the very bad is driven by the death drive and its dynamics, which always lead to the abolition of conflict through the summary elimination of one of its terms. Crimes of passion are an example of how the hyper-exaltation of the love object does not lead to its preservation but to its annihilation.

The suppression of love, previously described as a manic defense during the depressive position, has its roots in the danger posed by destructive impulses and persecutory anxiety. There are more psychotic moments, with a great split between love and hate, whereas, in neurotic moments, it is possible to manage destructiveness by repressing it. Predominantly psychotic moments harbor a paranoid-schizoid dynamic, while more neurotic moments exhibit a depressive dynamic[1].

The aspiration to be the creator of oneself and of the maternal breast, as well as the rejection of having been engendered, are the height of omnipotence and the denial of dependency. They signify a denial of one's own lineage and the refusal to belong to a lineage that preceded them. Rebelling against what has been instituted is an important ingredient in any creative and original action with transformative power; on the other hand, what is seen in psychosis is a massive refusal of filiation and the world created by ancestors, with the abolition and non-recognition of a reality shared with other human beings.

Now, let us see how these aspects are present in the analytic situation.

Envy in the analytical setting

At its core, envy is always directed at sources of life and creativity. As previously mentioned, "(…) envy is a most potent factor in undermining feelings of love and gratitude at their root, since it affects the earliest relation of all, that to the mother" (Klein, 1957/1975, p. 176). This last statement by Klein, made three years before her death, generated resistance within the English psychoanalytic community. However, it also opened a vast field of research into the negative therapeutic reaction, driven by a strong envy of the analyst's metaphoric and creative capacity.

The elaboration of envy and hatred is the fundamental task of analysis; but what exactly is this process of elaboration? From Klein's work, we can understand it as the repeated analysis of the anxieties and defenses linked to envy. Envy is the worst aspect of destructiveness, as it annihilates the internal good object, which is the foundation of psychic health. The analyst must persist, uncovering the darkest and most hidden feelings of envy that trace back to the primary maternal experience and refuse to come to light. The goal is to address the splitting processes and trace them back to their origin in order to dissolve them. It is essential, then, to analyze the envy felt toward the analyst, which leads the patient to relive the envy of the primary object.

There may frequently be destructive criticism of the analyst and everything they can offer through their interpretations. Such patients are incapable of expressing gratitude for any gift. As the popular saying goes, "that's just sour grapes…" Envy manifests through devaluing the other, as in the fable of the fox and the grapes, making it necessary to diminish the value of others' works and gifts. It becomes evident here the difficulty in valuing what is received – the subject turns their back on gratification and refuses what is offered. Envy "spoils" the enjoyment of good moments and the emergence of gratitude, which accompanies the ability to savor the exchange between two people, a situation that also occurs between analyst and analysand.

Indeed, envy can destroy and undermine all the analyst's work, turning it into something entirely devoid of value and meaning. The defenses against envy lead to indifference and increasingly devitalized forms of existence, in which love, desire, enthusiasm, and passion are either suppressed or absent.

In these circumstances, how is it possible to carry out the analytical work, which, according to Klein, consists of oscillating between moments of envy and moments of gratitude, among other dynamics? And how can one work through the splitting and other archaic defense mechanisms, such as omnipotence, denial, idealization, and devaluation?

Let us begin with an example to start reflecting on devaluation and defense against affective dependency and feelings of envy. If a patient feels they are being very destructive, they may try to lessen the guilt and persecution for damaging their objects out of envy by entering a state of confusion regarding their value. In other words, the patient might wonder: are these objects really good? Is the analyst really good, or a fraud? If the objects – including the analyst – lose value, the patient no longer needs to feel persecuted or guilty, resorting instead to splitting as a defense. Some analyses are interrupted during these moments of intense negative therapeutic reactions, requiring great skill from the analyst, who must allow themselves to be denigrated and attacked.

In more depressive and melancholic states, the devaluation of the object alternates with the subject's self-deprecation, as well as the devaluation of their gifts and achievements. Everything becomes devoid of importance and value – nothing is worthwhile. The feeling of impotence that the depressed patient projects onto the analyst is the way they find to destroy the analyst's potency, reducing it to nothing.

To spoil, to devalue – these are ways to avoid envy. A devalued object no longer needs to be envied. Some patients criticize an interpretation that had previously helped them, until nothing remains of it, sometimes not even the analysis itself. These defenses are activated in the dark recesses of the unconscious, and because they are so violent and radical, they cannot be undone quickly or omnipotently – in the same manner in which they were triggered.

For the analyst to work with these archaic anxieties and defenses, they must proceed slowly, with a great deal of availability and understanding toward the patient's envious attacks. Let us consider: if splitting exists to diminish the power of the bad object, or, in other words, to lessen the strength of highly unpleasant feelings of hatred, envy, and resentment, these feelings will not disappear unless they can gradually be integrated into the ego and the libidinal movements of the life instinct. Although we know that integration is never complete, splitting is the opposite movement, which allows for a radical, abrupt, and absolute elimination. What can we infer from this?

On the one hand, splitting and other schizoid defenses are radical defensive processes that produce an immediate result, aligned with the urgency and voracity of patients who operate from the paranoid-schizoid position and desire an immediate solution to their conflicts. What occurs, in reality, is the abolition of conflict, as splitting aims at the complete elimination of one of the poles of conflict. Transitioning from splitting to a process of integration involves a great deal of patient work. The analyst seeks to modify the functioning of this archaic ego that cannot tolerate pain, displeasure, or the presence of conflict and ambivalence.

Another important aspect is that envy stems from a predominance of oral and anal sadism. It is also part of the analyst's work to reduce this dynamic by creating a friendly, playful, and tolerant environment toward negative emotions, in order to facilitate their integration with the libido. It is necessary to reduce persecutory fears and analyze paranoid phantasies to allow for greater integration of love and hate. When hate and love are too dissociated from the ego, the patient may cover up their envy and destructiveness toward the analyst through defensive idealization.

The need to idealize, deny, and suppress emotions arises from the ego's inability to bear the tension of ambivalent affects, doubts, and hesitations. The patient then activates a rapid and radical defense mechanism, like splitting, which impoverishes the ego. In response to this, the analyst will invite the patient to the opposite dynamic, one of enrichment, showing that the negative affects and emotions they wish to eliminate will, in fact, be missed. If these emotions disappear, they will impoverish the patient psychically. In truth, it is necessary to increase the patient's confidence in their libidinal and loving aspects, which will counterbalance and integrate with their negative emotions[2].

The reader might ask: how does the analyst become this good object that fosters integration and growth? Fundamentally, it requires developing a deep understanding of the patient's state, who splits and loses access to their emotions. Distant hostility is their way of avoiding any risk or danger in contact with the other, which could generate attachment, dependency, and feelings of rejection. Thus, the splitting processes prevent the patient from coming into contact with themselves, leading them to become alienated and distant. Considerable parts of their personality are not accessible to them, which is why nothing makes sense – they hear the analyst but do not feel touched or affected. They do not feel present or like a real person. The interpretation must foster the patient's contact with themselves and their pain of living, which can then bring forth the arrival of a strong emotion. In some analytical situations, a powerful desire to cry may arise, almost as an eruption of something that had been under heavy containment.

With their attention, the analyst can probe the patient's anxieties that arise from the sensation of risk and danger in the contact with them, delicately touching upon these issues, and thus creating a reliable environment that accepts the patient's fears and uniqueness. The goal is to create conditions for the reestablishment of affective contact and the experience of an intimacy that does not intimidate or threaten but conveys security through the analyst's attentive, lively, and engaged presence.

The fundamental task of analysis is to expand the ego's capacity to endure and handle the impact of the Id and its drives, which give rise to helplessness, anxiety, pain, persecution, and guilt. The analyst engages in a process of acceptance, understanding, and transformation of the drives alongside the patient, increasing the patient's trust in their ability to endure and manage the Id, seen as a raw and blind force that can nevertheless be transformed into a creative force.

> In analysis we should make our way slowly' and gradually towards the painful insight into the divisions in the patient's self. This means that the destructive sides are again and again split off and regained, until greater integration comes about. As a result, the feeling of responsibility becomes stronger, and guilt and depression are more fully experienced. When this happens, the ego is strengthened, omnipotence of destructive impulses is diminished, together with envy, and the capacity for love and gratitude, stifled in the course of splitting processes, is released.
>
> (Klein, 1957/1975, p. 225)

Strengthening the ego means integrating and assimilating the impulses of the Id into it. A fragile ego is one that needs to dissociate these impulses from itself, either through repression (Freud) or splitting (Klein). The goal is not to subject the Id to the ego's adaptive power, but to enrich the ego by integrating the Id's drives, resulting in the liberation of emotional energies and an increased capacity for love, repair, and gratitude. To achieve this, it is necessary to reclaim and assume the destructive forces, especially envy, which greatly undermine the possibilities of positive experiences and satisfaction. Analysis should provide an environment of maximum tolerance toward the life of the drives, thereby promoting their integration into the ego.

Assimilation into the ego marks the moment when parental gifts can truly be appropriated and used by the ego. For this to occur, an early discrimination between good and bad experiences is required, accompanied by various processes of synthesis and integration between the two. The assimilation of these experiences into the ego allows it to claim its parental inheritance and become relatively autonomous.

> The insight gained in the process of integration makes it possible, in the course of the analysis, for the patient to recognize that there are potentially dangerous parts of his self. But when love can be sufficiently brought together with the split-off hate and envy, these emotions become bearable and diminish, because they are mitigated by love.
>
> (Klein, 1957/1975, p. 232)

When there are disturbances in the ability to work, create, and experience pleasure, one might hypothesize that this damage is being caused by the silent workings of envy. When unconscious envy is significant, the superego whispers the idea that it is not worth trying to repair the damage or create works that are branded as mediocre, leaving the individual paralyzed. Instead of guilt becoming a driving force for reparations, it turns into persecutory anxiety and a demand for punishment. How can this vicious cycle, stemming from self-diminishment, be reversed?

> The insight gained in the process of integration makes it possible, in the course of the analysis, for the patient to recognize that there are potentially dangerous parts of his self. But when love can be sufficiently brought together with the split-off hate and envy, these emotions become bearable and diminish, because they are mitigated by love.
>
> (Klein, 1957/1975, p. 233)

Our author believes that a deep sense of security can be obtained through contact with the mother or through analysis in contact with the analyst, stemming from the introjection of a whole, undamaged object. This is only possible when splitting has allowed for the discrimination between the good and bad. To work with states of fragmentation in analysis, it is necessary to let memories emerge through feeling, that is, the earliest memories preceding verbalization. This creates a new attitude toward old frustrations, thereby reducing the feeling of humiliation. A new capacity for enjoying the object is created, as envy prevents it from being used as a source of pleasure.

The analyst's work is to expand the ego's capacity to wait. By accepting uncomfortable states as stages of a process, the patient gradually learns to hold onto their impulses for longer, allowing for slower and more painful paths of transformation rather than immediately activating splitting and other radical defense mechanisms.

The analyst aims to dissolve the unconscious phantasies typical of envy, associated with oral, anal, and urethral sadism. The most primitive phantasies are those of extracting everything good from the mother and, conversely, ridding oneself by expelling into the mother's body everything with a negative connotation. These phantasies typically occur at a time when the child has a primitive ego, lacking the resources to think in words, yet feeling the need to evacuate their discomfort into the mother's body while voraciously emptying it of its good contents. The course of analysis, which aims to reach the earliest experiences and memories in feelings[3], allows these primitive experiences to enter a field of meaning and words, giving the patient a new position toward their archaic anxieties.

The introjection of the analyst as a good object creates a dynamic of integrations. Projective identifications decrease, and certain pleasant memories, previously buried, are recovered. Voracity and envy lose their power; hatred is mitigated by love, and the ego is strengthened by integrating negative emotions. The patient begins to feel gratitude, guilt, and responsibility.

It is necessary to reduce the patient's fear of their dimensions experienced as enemies and increase their trust in reparative and constructive forces, as well as their capacity for love. Negative emotions become less threatening if they can be integrated with love, as the risk of being overwhelmed by destructive aspects decreases, as does the pain in analysis. The patient can then regain the initiative to think their unthinkable thoughts, and their creativity grows, with the power to transform what seemed so threatening and unbearable into something viable[4].

Meltzer (1988) says that patients come to us to rid themselves of psychic pain, and what analysis offers is the development of a more effective, consistent, and expansive container to hold them. According to this understanding, we then transform, give meaning to, narrate, and repair life's inevitable pains through creative and aesthetic processes.

Notes

1 For further reading, see the text "Differentiation of the psychotic from the non-psychotic personalities" by Bion (1984).
2 The movie *Inside Out*, analyzed in Chapter 2 of this book, is a good example of these processes.
3 As Klein writes *memory in feelings*.
4 In the concepts of those who followed Klein, Winnicott, and Bion, the analyst must develop the qualities of the environmental mother, according to Winnicott – meaning the ability to provide *holding* and *handling*. According to Bion, the analyst should offer containment and reverie, to accommodate the patient's projective identifications.

References

Bion, R. W. (1959/1988). Attacks on linking. In: Spillus, E. B. (org.) *Melanie Klein today: Developments in theory and practice*. Vol. I. London: Routledge.
Bion, R. W. (1984). Differentiation of the psychotic from the non-psychotic personalities. In: *Second thoughts: Selected papers on psychoanalysis*. London: Karnac.
Klein, M. (1957/1975). Envy and gratitude. In: *Envy and gratitude and other works*. New York: The Free Press.
Meltzer, D. (1988). *The apprehension of beauty*. Scotland: The Clunie Press.

9 Projective identification

Technical developments

Elisa Maria de Ulhôa Cintra and
Marina F. R. Ribeiro

Klein observed that strong anxieties were present from the beginning of life, as previously mentioned. In the chronology of life, the first position is the paranoid-schizoid position; however, the depressive position was described in 1935 and 1940, and the paranoid-schizoid position in 1946. At that time, she also described, for the first time, another important concept: projective identification. This concept has had many developments and opened a broad field of investigation into the psychotic states of the mind, especially in the work of Herbert Rosenfeld, Hanna Segal, and Bion, psychoanalysts close to Klein in the 1940s and 1950s. The analysis of psychotic patients, within a strictly psychoanalytic framework, became possible through these psychoanalysts linked to the Kleinian circle.

Spillius[1] (2011, p. 8), when examining Klein's unpublished archives belonging to the M. Klein Trust, found that during 1946 and 1947, Klein was occupied with the paranoid-schizoid position and with the article she informally referred to as "my article on splitting". At no point did she name it "my article on projective identification", suggesting that the concept appeared unexpectedly.

Projective identification is one of the key concepts of the Kleinian theoretical-clinical framework that generated several other texts and discussions following its initial formulation. As Rocha Barros (2014, p. 16) highlights, "The fertility of an author can be measured by the number of new problems that arise after they are gone. These are people who not only provide fruitful answers but, above all, create a new field of inquiries[2]".

The clinical usefulness of projective identification is corroborated by the publication of various articles and books, as well as ongoing debates about the concept, not only among psychoanalysts of the English school (Quinodoz, 2012). Issues concerning changes in analytic technique are also part of the developments of projective identification, which emerge from Klein's clinical work and continually bring us back to the clinical practice. The potential of this concept was evidenced by the psychoanalysts who succeeded her, particularly those from her close circle: Bion, Segal, and Rosenfeld, who

DOI: 10.4324/9781003583035-10

demonstrated the breadth of projective identification in both theoretical and clinical dimensions.

Meltzer (1978) underscores the significance of two fundamental concepts – splitting and projective identification – by proposing that much of the research over the subsequent thirty years could be framed in terms of their phenomenology and implications.

Projective identification can be understood as an unconscious phantasy between analyst and analysand, which can have a more aggressive and expulsive, hence defensive, character; or a more communicative one. Splitting and projection mechanisms, in varying intensities, are always involved. To reach this formulation, a path was followed by several psychoanalytic theorists and clinicians, among them Bion, all belonging to the Kleinian circle. I will now briefly outline this trajectory.

In her 1946 text, Klein formulated projective identification as a defensive mechanism in response to paranoid-schizoid anxieties. It is a specific form of identification that involves the violent expulsion of parts of the *self* into the object, weakening the ego, and creating confusion and indistinction between subject and object. If the expulsion involves parts deemed bad, this will intensify the sense of persecution towards the object. If the projection of good parts predominates, this can either make object relations more loving – favoring the introjection of the good object and generating integration – or weaken the ego if the projection of good parts is excessive. In other words, when the projection of good parts is too great, the mother (and later other people) may become the ego ideal, fostering extreme dependency and impoverishing the ego, as all the good aspects are attributed to another and cannot be assimilated by the ego[3].

Klein (1946/1975) considers that "The processes of splitting off parts of the self and projecting them into objects are thus of vital importance for normal development as well as for abnormal object-relations". In the first explicit appearance of the concept – which had been inferred and germinating in earlier texts – Klein already recognized the normal and vital aspect of projective identification, something later emphasized by Bion (1959/1988 and 1962/1984).

In 1952, in "Some Theoretical Conclusions Regarding the Emotional Life of the Infant", Klein briefly observed the complementarity of projective and introjective identification processes. The ego becomes indistinguishable from the object; there is a projective and introjective amalgam of the ego and object (Baranger, 1981).

In her 1955 text, "On Identification", Klein, among other issues, comments on the non-pathological aspect of projective identification, drawing it closer to the concept of empathy. She discusses the functional aspects of splitting: if it occurs under the dominance of the good object, the split-off parts of the ego and the object can be recovered and brought closer. This differs from splitting under the dominance of the bad object, where fragmentation and dispersal of the object and the ego occur, and in this case, the parts may be lost and unre-coverable, leading to a process of ego depletion (Baranger, 1981).

In her 1957 text, "Envy and Gratitude", Klein postulates that envy is the *princeps* representative of the death drive. When excessive, it intensifies paranoid-schizoid anxieties, whose main defense mechanism is projective identification in its expulsive and violent form. She describes how massive projective identification leads to great confusion between *self* and object, as well as significant ego weakening and severe compromise of object relations.

Klein's (1946, 1952, 1955, and 1957) work on projective identification paved the way for Bion to reveal the complexity of the concept and its wide-ranging clinical applications. The pathological aspect of projective identifi-cation predominated in Kleinian texts, or perhaps we could say, prevailed in many of her readers and commentators. However, it was understood from a different angle in Bion's work: the non-verbal communication of mental states became more prominent.

In his 1959 article "Attacks on Linking", Bion reports that there is a normal degree of projective identification and that, associated with this, introjective identification constitutes the foundation upon which normal development rests, a point subtly indicated by Klein. In this article, Bion presents several clinical accounts, one of which describes how a patient split off his fears and deposited them in the analyst so that the analyst's mind could transform them, making them tolerable and then reintrojecting them into the patient's mind. In this situation, there is an opportunity for the patient to experience for the first time the emotional containment of his own anxieties, an opportunity that was likely previously denied by a mother who was mentally unavailable to hold and contain the infant's anxieties:

> Gratitude for the opportunity coexists with hostility to the analyst as the person who will not understand and refuses the patient the use of the only method of communication by which he feels he can make himself under-stood. Thus the link between patient and analyst, or infant and breast, is the mechanism of projective identification.
>
> (Bion, 1959/2014, p. 149)

Projective identification is understood as a link, with a communicative aspect, where the psychic qualities (regarding the containment of the baby's and the patient's anxieties) of the mother's and the analyst's minds are considered. This understanding expands upon Klein's original concept. The normal aspect, already present in Klein's work, is emphasized. Bion highlights the function of communicating mental states and considers the psychic conditions of the recipient of projective identification. Projective identification comes to be understood as a primordial link between baby and mother, and between ana-lyst and patient. This link, in Bion's 1959 text, relates to the mother's and the analyst's capacity to contain and transform projective identifications.

Bion (1959/1988) writes: "Projective identification [of the analysand] allows them to explore their own feelings within the personality of the analyst, which is strong enough to contain them[4]". Bion considers both environmental aspects and those stemming from aggression and primary envy. The origin of the disturbance is dual, both endogenous and exogenous, beginning with life itself. That is, a baby may have its phantasized attacks on the breast mitigated by the mother's capacity to contain and transform them, or not, in situations where this maternal capacity is insufficient or absent.

In the 1957 article, "Differentiation of Psychotic from the non-psychotic Personalities," Bion reports that even in patients where psychotic mechanisms predominate, we can still find situations in which the patient functions neurotically. Conversely, in non-psychotic patients, there may be moments of psychotic functioning. In projective identification where aggressive and expulsive aspects dominate, psychotic functioning prevails. In projective identification where communicative aspects stand out, we observe non-psychotic functioning. The degree of projection violence and extreme splitting are references for identifying psychotic or *borderline* functioning. There are different intensities of projective identification, and even in psychotic personalities, there is still a communicative aspect, while in non-psychotic personalities, splitting and projection also occur, though in milder forms.

In his 1962 article "A Theory of Thinking", Bion writes that the activity we know as "thinking" originally emerged as a procedure to discharge the psyche from increased stimuli, and that this mechanism was termed projective identification by Klein. Projective identification is an omnipotent phantasy in which undesirable or valuable parts of the psyche are dissociated and placed into the object. Bion notes that excessive projective identification results from two factors: the analyst's lack of containment to momentarily hold the patient's split-off parts, or an intense denial of reality on the part of the patient. The psychic qualities of the analyst's mind, particularly the capacity for containment, are fundamental – reflecting, retrospectively, the mother as the first object. In other words, the analyst must have the psychic conditions to tolerate being the depository of the patient's undesirable or valuable parts, serving as a container for the patient's anxieties.

Bion's understanding of projective identification is also that it is a basic activity of the human mind for communicating emotions, now considered at the origin of thinking. Beyond highlighting the fundamental aspect of human communication, Bion places the concept within the field of intersubjectivity. While in Klein's text projective identification predominantly reflects aspects of the internal, intrapsychic world, in Bion, the concept increasingly belongs to the interpersonal realm.

Projective identification, empathy, and countertransference

In 1959, Klein[5] stated in "Our Adult World and Its Roots in Infancy" that empathy would be a benign form of projective identification, involving "putting oneself in the other's shoes", differing from pathological forms of projective identification, in which there is greater disturbance at the boundaries between self and other, and more confusion of identities.

We can now consider the importance of the empathic attitude in the recently published Clinical Seminars on Melanie Klein's Technique, as commented on by John Steiner (2017).

From the beginning of Klein's clinical activity, and persistently in her clinical seminars, the issue of empathy is linked to an ever-present concern: that of capturing the patient's point of maximum anxiety: "(...) anxiety is like explosive material that can be managed in small amounts if it is handled with care" (Klein [1936] apud Steiner, 2017, p. 16). She also states in these clinical seminars held in 1936 at the British Psychoanalytical Society.

> However, the art of interpretation is only part of our work. We must keep in mind that another very essential part is to give full attention to the associations of the patient, to allow him to express his feelings, thoughts, fully; to pay full attention to this, to understanding fully the defences, and altogether to be as interested in his ego as we are in his unconscious. This implies that our interest could not and should not only be directed towards what we are going to interpret, because this should be based on the picture which we allow to emerge at his own pace. We have to keep a balance between the need of the patient to produce his material, to express his feelings and give full rope to that need. And we are thus confronted with the necessity to keep a balance between the time we are giving in an analytic session to this part of the work (which is in fact the fundament on which we base our interpretations) and the interpretations themselves.
>
> (Klein [1936] apud Steiner, 2017, pp. 15–16)

In this passage, we have a very vivid description of the analyst's empathic attitude, which is necessary for dealing with the "explosive material" of anxiety that needs to be managed in small quantities and with great care. It is anxiety itself, in its most heightened and archaic form, that demands empathy.

On the other hand, from very early on, Klein noticed the need that children had to project aggressive impulses of voracity and expressed an intense desire to control their own emotions and the feared emotions that could suddenly arise in others. An example of this appears in the case of Gerard, who "proposed to send it into the next room to carry out his aggressive desires on the father (...) This primitive part of the personality was in this case represented by the tiger" (Klein, 1927, p. 172).

The primitive part of the personality, manifested through oral, anal, urethral, and phallic drives, is linked to phantasies of seizing what is good and satisfying and eliminating what is bad and frustrating, in a dynamic that reflects the most basic processes of feeding and evacuation. It also encompasses the desire to cross the boundaries between self and other and the desire to know the interior of another's body and mind. The unconscious phantasy underlying projective identification, therefore, corresponds precisely to the belief that it is possible to cross these boundaries and rid oneself of aggression through projection. At the same time, these movements serve to communicate this frightening dimension to the analyst and to ask them to do something with that which is unbearable: it is a cry for help. The Gerard case was handled by Klein in the 1920s, anticipating what was later theorized.

Later, in the 1946 text on schizoid mechanisms, Klein introduced the term "projective identification", as mentioned before, to describe the tendency to rid oneself of everything that is aggressive and frightening. Early on, she noted that the most severe patients used this defense in an "excessive" or "massive" manner, while in other patients, projective identification did not seem to correspond to such an omnipotent belief that they could rid themselves of their aggression by controlling both their own psychic reality and that of others. Furthermore, a welcoming attitude in the environment allowed some of these beliefs to be transformed, leading patients to readmit the split-off and projected aspects into themselves.

Bion (1962/1984) points out that the expression "excessive projective identification", often found in Klein's texts, should be understood less as a description of the frequency with which it is employed and more in relation to the omnipotent and delusional quality of the belief underlying it. If the patient believes they have the magical power to control their psychic reality, they are more trapped in an illusion and may use the mechanism of projective identification excessively to refuse everything that destabilizes them. For example, the situation of being separated from their sources of nourishment, or to avoid admitting their needs and dependencies, to deny their own envy and resentment. It is, after all, a primitive defense mechanism that attempts to annihilate any and all situations of helplessness, and psychic reality itself, in its violent and frightening aspects.

The most pathological projective identifications are those in which there is a strong rejection of these harsh realities, as they are experienced as unacceptable, making it difficult to relinquish the omnipotent belief of having rid oneself of "that abominable psychic reality". This entire process leads to a greater distortion of the perception of the external and internal worlds; however, rejecting these realities brings immediate relief.

In projective identifications with a more communicative nature, the patient may experience projective identification as if it were a transitional phenomenon, serving as a bridge to a subsequent moment in which, after being denied, the impulses can be readmitted, recovering a significant part of the drive and the lost identifications. We can think of it as a game of make-believe, as if the patient were saying: "Here, take this part of me and pretend it's yours for a while, then give it back to me".

The greater the aspiration to omnipotently control psychic reality and remain in a state of fusion with the object, the greater the anxiety and fear, and the more imprisoning the mechanism becomes. The more the projection of aspects of the patient's psychic reality onto the analyst (or the mother, in the early stages) can be welcomed and contained by the environment, the more it will enter the symbolic field and acquire the power to become a game and a communication.

When postulating the mechanisms of projection and introjection, particularly the mechanism of projective identification, Melanie Klein did not ignore the presence of different states of undifferentiation between subject and object, both in psychic constitution and in the analytic process. One of the achievements of maturation is precisely reaching increasingly sophisticated levels of separation between self and other, while recognizing that this coexists with moments and states of relative undifferentiation, in successive cycles.

I believe moments of undifferentiation can be experienced as transitional phenomena when they are welcomed by the environment, and can enter the realm of metaphor through play, humor, make-believe games, and the infinite forms of containment and symbolization that culture offers. Following Winnicott's (1971) inspiration, we can think of moments of undifferentiation and communicative projective identification, when met with empathy, as wave-forming cycles, alternating until reaching moments of greater differentiation, that is, a process of transitionality.

Bion (1959/2003) published his theory on "Attacks on linking" based on work with a patient who seemed to have never had, before the analytic encounter, the opportunity to direct their projective identifications toward a sufficiently welcoming environment.

> (...) There were sessions which led me to suppose that the patient felt there was some object that denied him the use of projective identification. (...) the patient felt that parts of his personality that he wished to repose in me were refused. When the patient strove to rid himself of fears of death which were felt to be too powerful for his personality to contain he split off his fears and put them into me, the idea apparently being that if they were allowed to repose there long enough they would undergo modification by my psyche and could then be safely reintrojected.
>
> (Bion, 1959/2003, p. 96)

Bion raises the following hypothesis: could it be that this patient's mother felt great impatience toward the baby's anxieties and wondered: what is wrong with this child? Therefore, she was unable to provide containment for the baby's anxieties. The author writes:

> From the infant's point of view, she should have taken into her, and thus experienced, the fear that the child was dying. It was this fear that the child could not contain. (...) An understanding mother is able to experience the feeling of dread, that this baby was striving to deal with by projective identification, and yet retain a balanced outlook. This patient had had to deal with a mother who could not tolerate experiencing such feelings and

reacted either by denying the ingress, or alternatively by becoming a prey to the anxiety which resulted from the introjection of the infant's feelings.

(Bion, 1959/2003, pp. 96–97)

Reverie is a maternal function, and also an analytic function, which denotes a state of openness to receiving the emotions and projections arising from the baby and/or the patient. Bion considers that it is necessary to receive, contain, and process the patient's projective identifications through a work of transformation that captures sensory impressions and all pre-verbal communications – the so-called beta-elements – converting them into alpha-elements, which are fit to enter a process of symbolization and may eventually be verbalized. The analyst's experience of *reverie* offers great relief to the patient and reveals the analyst's empathic capacity to attune to the patient's still-un-symbolized aspects.

The analyst's empathic capacity helps the patient also develop an empathic quality toward what is enigmatic and uncomfortable, contributing to the formation of their alpha-function and the psychic apparatus. Bion considers that the analysand acquires psychic qualities by sharing the psychic qualities of the analyst's mind. For Bion, the fear the analyst feels toward their own feelings is an obstacle to understanding the patient's communications, preventing the establishment of empathy.

From this perspective, the central aspect of analytic empathy would be the existence of an analyst capable of *reverie*, which is built through projective identifications between them and the patient, so that both can understand what is happening in the emotional experience of the analytic session. Empathy would be a benign form of projective identification, a "putting oneself in the other's shoes," or rather, using the ability to perceive oneself, implanting it in the other, to metaphorically intuit what is happening with them.

A scholar of the work of Bion, Grotstein (1981), suggests that through interpretations, the analyst invites the patient to empathize with their own sense of helplessness and repressed, split-off parts. He passionately underscores the need for all people, especially patients, to share their most primal experiences, using projective identification in a communicative and empathic way. An anguished patient can only feel understood by the analyst when they experience, in some way, those emotions that the patient cannot verbalize. We project our experiences, deeply hoping that the other person will understand what we cannot communicate, seeking relief by being comprehended. True relief comes only when we are convinced that the other person now concretely holds our experience emotionally.

Inspired by Grotstein (1981), we can assert that the empathic use of projective identification ultimately depends on the one receiving it and their capacity for *reverie*. The greater the analyst's empathy and metaphorical ability, as well as their capacity to detach from their emotions in order to understand them, the greater their ability to transform the patient's projective identifications into communications that can enrich both. Following Bion and his successors, such as Grotstein, Bollas, Ogden, and Ferro, this defense mechanism has been understood in its intersubjective dimension, as previously mentioned. Most contemporary Kleinians believe that the projective identifications of patients must be contained and processed by the analyst so that they can be returned to the patient in a way that facilitates the elaboration process.

In fact, Klein's description of projective identification followed her tendency to understand the psyche and its mechanisms with an emphasis on the intrapsychic dimension. Like Freud, she remained skeptical about the use of countertransference to understand the patient.

According to Etchegoyen and Minuchin (2014), Klein provided us with the main tool for understanding countertransference – projective identification – meaning that she opened the field for the concept of countertransference, even if she did not acknowledge this and strongly opposed Heimann's ideas.

In the 1950s, Paula Heimann proposed a broader use of countertransference. In his book *The Shadow of the Object*, Bollas (2018) reminds us that until that point, in 1950, it was assumed that the person speaking in analysis was the patient, from the perspective of their conscious or unconscious discourse. Without ceasing to listen to the patient's free associations, Paula Heimann decided to open her listening to an array of subjective voices from different psychic strata: "Who is speaking, at this moment, through this patient?" and "To whom is he addressing his words?"

> (...) Heimann realized that at one moment the analysand was speaking to the mother, anticipating the father, or reproaching, exciting, or consoling a child – the child self of infancy, in the midst of separation at age two, in the oedipal phase, or in adolescence (...) The patient's narrative was not simply listened to in order to hear the dissonant sounds of unconscious punctuation (...) The British analyst would also analyze the shifting subjects and others that were implied in the life of the transference.
>
> (Bollas, 2018, p. 13)

The simultaneous presence of a multitude of subjects within a single person invited the analyst to engage more deeply in their listening work, thus initiating what we now call an implicated analyst.

This implication – without denying the necessary reserve (Figueiredo, 2009) and abstinence of the analyst – leads the analyst to expand their porosity and ability to be physically and emotionally affected by what the patient says, while also summoning their most archaic bodily memories and their own personal history and analysis.

The goal is to "listen with the whole body[6]" (Cintra, 1998), to be willing to be used by the patient as a sufficiently acoustic environment to resonate with and acknowledge what is being communicated. The analyst's capacity for empathy and the quality of their presence have gradually become more important, and we must increasingly think about what this quality of presence means.

To be truly present to the other requires a capacity for *reverie* – dreaming the other from the experience of having been dreamed by someone else. It stems from a real ability to see, listen to, and feel the other, while also requiring a negative capability (Cintra, 2017); that is, the analyst must withdraw from their own imaginary and the pull of their narcissistic desires, even as they inhabit them. Is this possible?

Perhaps it is somewhat idealistic to imagine an analyst who can hear the polyphony of voices and subjects within a single subject. However, what can be done are simple movements in this direction. To begin, a movement of letting go of one's technical and theoretical certainties, allowing the patient's participation to correct the analyst's interpretations and constructions. Perhaps the most important thing is simply the desire to stop judging, to stop understanding everything. This, along with training in polyphonic listening, can foster the analytic attitude. The insights gained in the analyst's own analysis are what make them empathic toward the patient they are listening to today.

Since the late 1950s, British analysts have begun monitoring projective identifications in the field of transference and countertransference. Patients discovered that analysts had the ability to receive, welcome, decode, and name experiences from a time before the acquisition of verbal language, from the world of the child, using their countertransferential reactions. And this was quite revolutionary.

With Klein, we learned that anxieties at their peak intensity are explosive material; they demand the analyst's empathic capacity. And with Bion, we learned that the more primitive and intense the emotion, the greater the need for two minds to handle the event. This requires the presence of a fearless analyst, one who has walked the paths of their own *childhood* and who has been heard, in their own analysis, through *reverie* and empathy.

Notes

1 Some ideas developed in this section are present in the chapter A Conceptual Reflection Between Projective Identification and Enactment (Ribeiro, M. F. R., 2017).
2 TN: Translation provided by the translator.
3 Segundo Hinshelwood (Spillius, 2011): "Klein does not use the term 'ego' in as precise a way as Freud came to do with his structural model of the ego, the id and the superego. She often uses 'ego' interchangeably with 'self'".
4 TN: Translation provided by the translator.
5 Some of the ideas in this section are present in the text "Empathy, Projective Identification, and Reverie: Listening to the Unheard in Trauma Therapy" (Cintra, 2017).
6 TN: Translation provided by the translator.

References

Baranger, W. (1981). *Posição e objeto na obra de Melanie Klein*. Porto Alegre: Editora Artes Médicas Sul LTDA. (translation: Position and object in the works of Melanie Klein).

Barros, E. M. R. (2014). Prefácio. In: *Leituras criativas: ensaios sobre obras analíticas seminais / Thomas H. Ogden*. São Paulo: Editora Escuta. (Translation: Foreword. In: Creative readings: Essays on seminal analytic works / Thomas H. Ogden).

Bion, W. R. (1957/2014) The differentiation of the psychotic from the non-psychotic personalities. In: *The complete works of W. R. Bion*. London: Karnac. Edited by Chris Mawson and editorial consultancy by Francesca Bion.

Bion, W. R. (1959/2003). Attacks on linking. In: Spillus, E. B. (org.) *Melanie Klein today: Developments in theory and practice*. Vol. I. London: Brunner-Routledge.

Bion, W. R. (1962/1984). A theory of thinking. In: *Second thoughts*. London: Karnac.

Bion, W. R. (1967/2014). Attacks on linking. In: *Second thoughts*: Selected papers on psycho-analysis. In: *The complete works of W. R. Bion*. London: Karnac. Edited by Chris Mawson and editorial consultancy by Francesca Bion.

Bollas, C. (2018). *The shadow of the object: Psychoanalysis of the unthought known*. London; New York: Routledge.

Cintra, E. M. U. (1998). Escutar com o corpo inteiro. Percurso Revista de Psicanálise, Ano XI, n. 21-2, p.129–131. (Translation: Listening with the Whole body).

Cintra, E. M. U. and others (2017). Empatia, identificação projetiva e reverie: escutar o inaudível na clínica do trauma. In: *Para além da contratransferência – O analista implicado*. São Paulo: Zagodoni. (Translation: Empathy, projective identification, and reverie: listening to the inaudible in trauma therapy. In: *Beyond countertransference – The involved analyst*).

Etchegoyen, H. and Minuchin, L. (2014). *Seminarios de introducción a su obra*. Buenos Aires: Ediciones Biebel. (Translation: Seminars on introduction to her work).

Figueiredo, L. C. (2009). *As diversas faces do cuidar – novos ensaios de psicanálise contemporânea*. São Paulo: Escuta. (Translation: The various faces of caring – New essays in contemporary psychoanalysis).

Grotstein, J. S. (1981). *Splitting and projective identification*. New York: Jason Aronson.

Heimann, P. (1950). On counter-transference. *International Journal Psycho-Analysis*, 31:81–84.

Klein, M. (1927/1975). Criminal tendencies in normal children. In: *Love, guilt and reparation and other works*. New York: Dell Publishing Co.

Klein, M. (1935/1975). A contribution to the theory of intellectual inhibition states. In: *Love, guilt and reparation and other works*. New York: Dell Publishing Co.

Klein, M. (1936/1975). Weaning. In: *Love, guilt and reparation and other works*. New York: Dell Publishing Co.

Klein, M. (1940/1975). Mourning and its relation to manic-depressive states. In: *Love, guilt and reparation and other works*. New York: Dell Publishing Co.

Klein, M. (1946/1975). Notes on some schizoid mechanism. In: *Envy and gratitude and other works*. New York: The Free Press.

Klein, M. (1952/2018). Some theoretical conclusions regarding the emotional life of the infant. In: *Developments in psychoanalysis*. London & New York: Routledge Edited By Paula Heimann, Susan Isaacs, Melanie Klein, Joan Riviere.

Klein, M. (1955/1975). On identification. In: *Envy and gratitude and other works*. New York: The Free Press.

Klein, M. (1957/1975). Envy and gratitude. In: *Envy and gratitude and other works*. New York: The Free Press.

Klein, M. (1959/1975). Our adult world and its roots in infancy. In: *Envy and gratitude and other works*. New York: The Free Press

Quinodoz, J.-M. and others (2012). Projective identification in contemporary French-language psychoanalysis. In: *Projective identification – The fate of a concept.* London; New York: Routledge.

Spillus, E. B. and others (2011). *The new dictionary of Kleinian thought.* London; New York: Routledge.

Steiner, J. (2017). *Lectures on technique by Melanie Klein.* London: Routledge.

Winnicott, D. W. (1971). Transitional objects and transitional Phenomena. In: *Playing and reality.* London: Tavistock Publication.

10 Reflections on and beyond Melanie Klein

Elisa Maria de Ulhôa Cintra

In this chapter we present three texts by Elisa Maria de Ulhôa Cintra, which were previously published in journals. The first, "Mourning and Melancholia: a Reflection on Purifying and Destroying" is inspired by Freud's Mourning and Melancholia, and it raises the following question: what enables us to begin the mourning process and what is it that leads to the impossible mourning of melancholia? The violent self-recriminations of melancholia are illustrated by the film *Shutter Island*, by Martin Scorcese (2009). Melanie Klein's theory of the primitive superego and Winnicott's theory of our capacity for concern for the other are also evoked here.

The second piece, "The Third Bank of the River", is a reflection upon violence, hatred, and intolerance as viewed through the prism of the September 11, 2001 terrorist attacks in the USA. In addition to Klein's psychoanalytical frame of reference, we also draw upon some of Levinas' ideas. The metaphor of the "third bank of the river" is taken from the short story of the same name by Guimarães Rosa, and it is used as a tool through which to consider parenting as an activity of being, giving being to, bringing to be, and of letting the other be.

The third piece, "On the Feeling of Solitude", is based on Winnicott's "The Capacity to Be Alone" (1958), which probes the roots of this capacity, and the conditions that make it possible. The capacity to be alone is grounded in the relationship to one's mother – and herein lies a paradox: being alone demands the presence and relaxed company of someone else, by your side, absently available, someone with whom you can have contact at any time, whether in outer reality or in the virtual reality of your inner world.

Mourning and melancholia: a reflection on purifying and destroying

Human subjectivity is a sheaf of different temporalities. Life unfolds in transformations; the gradually shrinking exterior disappears and gives rise to an interior construct, a bundle of conscious and unconscious memories, some recent, others distant. Mourning for the childhood or adolescent body, for first loves, first homes, or cities we have lived in is all part of a psychic process on

DOI: 10.4324/9781003583035-11

which psychological and physical health depends. What enables the onset of mourning and what leads to the impossible mourning of melancholia? What sends the work of Eros into such a tailspin that the deobjectalizing dynamic of Thanatos can predominate? These are the questions that guide me through the sea of ideas that has emerged over the last hundred years out of the works of Freud, Melanie Klein, Winnicott, and others. The idea is to listen to what these authors have to say about mourning and melancholia in order to draw out the most fertile overlaps between their works, and the roots and ramifications of each in the other.

I think the self-reproaches of melancholia need to be grasped through accounts that evince the pain and the virulence of an imaginary designed to purify and destroy through mechanisms that exclude everything that has become intolerable. The film *Shutter Island*,[1] by Scorsese, serves as an example of just this tragic outcome, in which past events prove too terrible to process. In melancholia, when reason has become delirious, the order issued by the primitive Superego is decisive: purify and destroy. Purify, that is, the attribution of the negative quality, separating it entirely from the positive quality; divide the I into a judge that believes himself all-knowing, and a judged who is crushed under the weight of its damning asseverations. After that, all that remains to do is reduce oneself to the most abject creature in the world under a hail of reproaches.

A comparable process, given the level of violence directed towards the other, is visible in the various fundamentalisms of the 20th and 21st Centuries, and the genocides they spawned. The desire to elucidate some of the mechanisms responsible for total war[2] led me to reread Freud's Mourning and Melancholia (Freud, 1917) and draw some reflections on melancholic madness.

Historical background

For some years, between 1911 and 1921 at least, the theme of melancholia was a recurrent feature in the correspondence and meetings of psychoanalysts. Freud started writing Mourning and Melancholia in 1914, with the outbreak of the First World War (shocking for the indiscriminate violence directed toward all enemies, whether military or civilian), but ended up being published only in 1917. Its gestation was long and involved many peer discussions.

At this point in his work, Freud was taking the reader through the enigmas of child sexuality toward the functioning of the I. Abraham (1924/1979) makes the significant contribution of connecting melancholia to the oral-sadistic and anal-sadistic phases. At first, Freud resisted placing so much emphasis on sadism, but he ended up agreeing with Abraham. In 1914, he added a note to his Three Essays (1905), including the oral-sadistic stage alongside "primordially libidinal sucking".

In the oral-sadistic phase, the way in which the loved object is appropriated all but erases its "objectal" facet, leaving only the narcissistic aspect. In what manner can the object be in the service of the I, if the I wants to devour it, where it is lovable, and expel it, where it is detestable? One way or another, the object remains in the service of the ego, to be consumed or expelled, and so as both an oral and anal object at one and the same time. Delicious or disgusting, retained or expelled, the connection is at once extremely intense and fragile! The intensity derives from the idealization (and de-idealization) it carries, the "invention" of the other as per some narcissistic script, and from the way it attracts all the libido to be devoured, expelled, or entirely confused with the other or with the Ideal. The fragility, on the other hand, resides in the fact that all it takes to shatter the object into a thousand pieces is for it to stray just a little from the imaginary script created for it. And around the resulting ruins, skirting the fringes of the destruction, surge scathing hatred, disappointment, resentment, and rancor. Freud's reference to narcissistic object-choice (the process described above) shows that he was still wrangling with the issue of narcissism and the Ideals of the I he had recently developed in "On Narcissism: An Introduction" (Freud, 1914 and would pursue further in "Denial" (1925)). However, even before Abraham's insistence on the importance of sadism to any elucidation of melancholia, Freud had already revealed the intuition that hatred plays a vital role in this state:

> Hostile impulses against parents (a wish that they should die) are also an integrating constituent of neuroses. They come to light consciously as obsessional ideas. In paranoia the worst feature of delusions of persecution (pathological distrust of rulers and monarchs) corresponds to these hostile impulses against parents. These impulses are repressed at periods when compassion for the parents is aroused – at times of their illness or death. On such occasions it is a manifestation of mourning to reproach oneself for their death (so-called melancholia) or to punish oneself in a hysterical fashion, through the medium of the idea of retribution, with the same states [of illness] that they have had.[3]

Freud always creates a sort of syzygy between the healthy and pathological facets of a psychic process. As such, melancholia emerges as the pathological form of mourning. Conversely, the withdrawal into oneself of all invested libido as we see in narcissism is the unhealthy "version" of the dream process, when the libido washes back over our mnemic traces and the remembrance of "childhood". In this chapter, as the states of mourning and melancholia are unpacked, the reader will continuously hear the same question: what makes mourning possible (healthy), and impossible (pathological)? Since Freud, a century of writing has striven to answer this very question. Melanie Klein and Winnicott both built conceptions around that core, as did Nicolas Abraham, Maria Torok, Pierre Fedida, and many others besides, each of whom addressed the enigma of mourning in his or her own way.

The characteristics of melancholia and mourning in Freud

From the outset, Freud offered a precise description of melancholia as a profound dejection, the cessation of all interest in the outside world, the loss of the capacity to love, inhibition of all activity, and a decreased sense of self-esteem. All of that, for Freud, is also found in mourning, with the exception of decreased self-regard.

Mourning is considered here in terms of movement, passage; while melancholia is an impasse, where everything grinds to a halt: the object is gone and the ego condemns itself to no longer being or doing anything. The shadow of the object falls across the I and immobilizes it. Seeing itself thus, judged and condemned, the ego drags itself through a lengthy inertia, mired in despair. The feeling of inferiority that comes with it crushes every desire to move on. The sensation of being unable to be creates an enclave within the ego in which love and work are no longer possible and the aspects of grief – dejection, loss of interest in the world, numbness – become protracted, eternal, unending.

The process of mourning, on the other hand, kindles its own way forward, a will to work through the morass. But there's a whole other sense of "wading through" here, one that sends the mourner down the wild and meandering trails of gone time so that the past can be left in the past and a new future may open up ahead. No-one conducts this process, rather we are conducted by it; mourners must narrate their own lives to themselves and to attentive listeners, because an untold life is no life at all.

The idea of the work speaks to process, movement, the beginning of a temporal dynamic, the transformation of the lived; accepting loss, change, the facticity of destiny. The ancients used to speak of Amor fati (love of fate), which requires that we accept and learn to live with the reality of death, separation, loss, and lack.

Early on, Freud's readers, such as Abraham, Ferenczi, Jones, Melanie Klein, Winnicott, and others realized that the psychic apparatus exists, above all else, to metabolize the lived, let it pass on, be forgotten, itself a precondition of any future remembering. Letting the past be past and the ability to dream, these are the two Freudian pillars of mental health. We must dream the past, bring it to life, both present and future. After all, is that not the work the analyst and patient do together?

I look at subjectivity as a sheaf of heterogeneous temporalities that comprise and oppose each other, creating conflict, synthesis, contradiction, and paradox. Among the impasses created by experience, it is important to find intersections, short-cuts, passageways; otherwise, we end up trapped in the enclave of melancholia. Pontalis (1988) reveals the intimate intertwining of dreaming and mourning: the need to dream loss and death. When the other disappears, we feel incapable of continuing to love, and the flow of our love risks souring to hate or resentment. This is because, on the infantile level, the absence of the other becomes abandonment, a rejection we rail against…and hate. But we can make that object present again in dream…

> Is the most intolerable feature of loss the losing from sight which it involves? Does that mean the absolute withdrawal of love from the other and the instilling, within ourselves, of the restlessness of an essential fragility: that of not being able to love the invisible? First of all, we must be able to see. Not just see, but see first, and to be able to placate the inner anguish this absence incites, insuring that the loved object is entirely visible to the eye, and that it reflects us in our very identity. After all, why do we dream if not to see, every night, what has disappeared to us (worlds, places, people, faces), so as to confirm their permanence and try to reconcile the ephemeral and the eternal?
>
> (Pontalis, 1988/1991, p. 205)

In a certain sense, in mourning it is possible to overcome the loss and, with time, begin to feel interested in people and places again, in new faces; there's a rebirth of investment in the object, of world-directed libido. In melancholia, there is loss of self-respect, an undermining of the self and the other, the ego becomes impoverished and empty. Freud recalled Prince Hamlet here, and we are invited to read Shakespeare's tragedy whilst considering the dynamic of melancholia (Kristeva, 1999, Cintra, 2001). Once that sense of abandonment takes hold in melancholia, it is intolerable, but keeps being reprised nevertheless, over and over. There's a compulsion towards repetition – the Ego identifies with the Superego. The Ego splits in two: on one hand, there's identification with the abandoner, who says "I left you because you are worthless". And that severe criticism is leveled at the other side of the Ego, which feels abandoned, reduced to the condition of having been rejected. The act of abandoning involves more than leaving or disappearing, and can unfold on a daily basis in various other chronic gestures: disapproval, disdain, discrediting. Abandonment expresses the withdrawal of love and moral approval more completely than does simple physical separation; we're in the realm of value judgements here, Ideals, beliefs, the loss of the Superego's love, and of love full stop.

Two people might actually live together, yet cast the shadow of abandonment on each other the whole time, a situation that will see both of them fall sick. Freud teaches us to see that the main question is not death or the separation of people, but the hatred, revolt, and recrimination that emerges once the love has gone. The event of abandonment occupies the whole psychic scene, like an open wound, and it sucks all the libido toward itself, leading to dejection, ceased interest in the outside world, the inhibition of all activity and the loss of capacity to love. Love becomes hatred over having been abandoned and through the desire to abandon, meaning the object becomes, at the same time, the ideal/sadistic ego and the degenerate/masochistic ego. The dynamism that sets in is the oral-sadistic and anal-sadistic stage, and the I is treated as an oral object to be devoured and spat out and a fecal object to be retained and expelled without the slightest thought. The ego-object becomes the ego-abject.

Below are some lines from Hamlet's first soliloquy, in which, before reproaching himself, he disdains nature, his mother, and the human condition for the weeds that overrun them, giving rise to the desire for "self-slaughter".

> O, that this too too solid flesh would melt
> Thaw and resolve itself into a dew!
> Or that the Everlasting had not fix'd
> His canon 'gainst self-slaughter! O God! God!
> How weary, stale, flat and unprofitable,
> Seem to me all the uses of this world!
> Fie on't! ah fie! 'tis an unweeded garden,
> That grows to seed; things rank and gross in nature
> Possess it merely. That it should come to this!
>   (Shakespeare, 1603, Act I, Sc 2)

Devastating feeling of guilt: archaic Superego and the Scorcese film *Shutter Island*, a story told from the perspective of insanity

The suffering of melancholia has not yet been sufficiently explored. Some clinical cases, films, and books can help us obtain a better sense of the violence of the pain it causes, which can lead to suicide or psychic death. Love is successively transformed into hate, and into the desire to kill or die, and that murderous, suicidal hatred plunges the sufferer into the most devastating guilt. It's the feeling of dark, persecutory guilt of the Erinyes that gnaws and shreds. A guilt that does not know how to cry or beg forgiveness, nor to embrace and make amends.

Those hoping to understand the violence of unbearable, madness-inducing guilt, strong enough to block out reality and drive one into isolation, should watch the Martin Scorsese film *Shutter Island*.[4] The island of the title is "shutter than shut", a prison in and of itself from which no-one can escape, like a circle closing in on itself, and shutting out an even more unbearable reality and unspeakable pain.

Freud (1910) had a term for this island on which the psychotic self-isolates, away from contact with shared reality. He called it "neoreality". The insanity of Daniels, the main character in *Shutter Island*, displays some elements of melancholia and others of paranoia: he lives in fear and constant distrust of others. His hallucinations reveal the unadulterated violence of his imaginary, constantly playing out in war flashbacks and appearances of his dead wife and children. To defend himself against so much pain, he builds a delirium that is, in itself, an attempt to impose order on the chaos, but in doing so it traps him inside a closed system.

In the film, the cliff-girded island sits surrounded by ocean, the stumps of storm-snapped trees testifying to the metaphorical tempests that rage in the inner world of madness. "God loves violence", says one of the characters, a soldier who is the very embodiment of all that is most detestable in an authority figure. We will see later how the director uses the resources of nature's fury and the real and imagined sadism of the island's medical and military personnel in building the dark and solitary labyrinth of mental illness.

However, before we return to the film, we will first look at how Freud renders the solitary island of melancholia. In "Mourning and Melancholia" (1917), Freud examines the Ego, the cleaving of the Ego, and the Ego divided into the voices of the oppressor and that of the oppressed, elements that lie at the root of the idea of the cruel and archaic Superego. The I begins to function as a stage, and the idea of the scene, spun by the analysis of dreams and fantasies, spills onto that stage as characters and voices. Who are these characters (the identifications) that will play the scenes? How many identifications go into an ego? What are these voices, the presences and absences that form the ego? The I begins to emerge as a polyphony, a conjunct of solos, duets, trios, and silences. It's easy to see here the origin of Freud's theories of object relations, because these voices create together a diverse range of dynamisms of unity, opposition, war and peace. Future internal objects.

The critical agency, or Superego, for example, will be a jumble of different loves and hatreds transformed into identifications. It will be a combination of external events with different interpretations edited by an ego with its own threshold for pain, trauma, frustration, and abandonment. After abandonment, the love for a highly-idealized object converts into a series of pure identifications, forming a severe critical agency that condemns and attacks the ego, which is too fragile to tolerate a traumatic situation. The stage is set for the advent of melancholia, which would later come to be seen as the perfect culture for the death instinct.

A cloister or enclave forms: on one hand, the love felt for the object cannot be abandoned, but becomes radicalized as pure love, pure hate. Pure states do not mix, so the polarization that emerges is radical, with no blending allowed. The hatred becomes extreme, steeled by pain, dejection and abandonment, and out of that comes an unbearable feeling of guilt.

In *Shutter Island* we see an oscillation between the desire for, and fear of, revenge, the guilt Daniels feels for not having protected his children from their mother's madness, and a tremendous anguish: Daniels is afraid that he will be unable to live in a reality soaked in so much death. His recent psychic reality is increasingly brutal, given the sum (and multiplication) of the wounds of the past, making mourning impossible. "Which would be worse – to live as a monster, or to die as a good man?", asks Daniels, before, at the end of the story, opting for a lobotomy.

Let me briefly run through the film's plot: the protagonist arrives on the island as a Federal Marshal tasked with investigating the escape of a dangerous murderer, an inmate at this "shutter than shut", cliff-walled asylum for the criminally insane, which can be reached or left only by ferry.

And that's how Daniels and his partner, Chuck, arrive: by ferry, slowly emerging out of the nebulous white that fills the screen. From the very first scenes, as they approach this sinister place, blanketed in sea-fog, we are plunged into a misty blur-zone between sanity and madness. Daniels, known to be a brave and violent man, is seasick and terrified of the water. His strength disappears before the deadly power of the ocean, pivotal in the dissolution and destruction of his past life.

The four elements, earth, air, fire, and water, seem to be key to the story, which rolls out a tale of horror and suspense that includes blazes, drownings, nightmares brought on by dripping leaks, sombre corridors and matches struck to light fires or the cigarettes he fears contain hallucinogenic substances. Daniels is persecuted by everyone, and becomes their persecutor in return. He is a well of persecutory angst. The director conjures a noir atmosphere that is a little caricatural, perhaps as a device to mark the change in perception (forms, times, memories) that occurs in madness, heightened by a sense of suspense and menace created by the musical score. Caught between hallucination, delirium, sight, and touch, Daniels and the viewer find themselves in a strange neoreality. Nobody can help them. Who or what can they trust? Their own eyes? Other people's words? The director plays with the overly dark and excessively bright, to the point of blinding us with the difference between the imagined and perceived.

Early on, we begin to ask ourselves whether Daniels is there on official business or in search of vengeance, or, perhaps, out of guilt and remorse. The viewer is transported to a borderland between love and hate, guilt and vengeance, madness and sanity. When the film ends, we still can't really be sure if it was all just delirium or hallucination. The director knows full well just how many labyrinths it takes to dismantle an ego. And he leaves us there – amid the ruins, among chunks of dead and wounded humanity languishing in the snow – scared to death of going mad as well. Watching this film means experiencing the vertigo of madness; we feel all our references of reality waver.

At the end, as the credits roll, a song plays from the visceral depths of a singer's soul: "What if my life is like the dust?" (Mirage, dream, hallucination?). Or "What good is love that no one shares?" The song is called "Bitter Earth"[5], and there could have been no better way to close the film than with that wounded voice, which tears at the listener from the inside.

The question "And what if my life is like the dust?" recalls one of the scenes in the film, in which Daniels hugs his wife, Dolores: it's all a dream, because she is dead, but his hallucination is so very real. He wants her back, he wants to hold her, and he's sure that, even though she died in a fire, he can embrace her now with passion and longing. But he can't. When she turns, her back is a caved-in hole of scorched embers, and when he wraps his arms around her, blood and water gush through the fingers of his linked hands. When he holds her more tightly, she crumbles into ash. Bitter Earth. The lyrics to the song continue to resound, and we understand that his memories of war are telling us that Daniels was forced to kill, and kill many. He killed to survive and did survive, but his ego was rent down the middle by horror and necessity: on one side, his values, compassion and desire to live and be happy; on the other, horror, and the need to survive it.

After the war, his denial of Dolores's madness and his guilt for not protecting his children shred his ego even more. "And what if my life was like the dust?". Dust and ash, a bitter earth. The hallucination is Daniel's life: turning to dust and ash around a body that is no longer there.

However, his fixation on his wife cannot be abandoned. That would mean letting her go, letting the past be past; various voices in his hallucination implore him to let Dolores go – the condition for any potential exit from the closed system in which he has jailed himself. She, herself, appears to him in dreams and visions and begs him to let her depart. But his strange love for her, which he cannot relinquish, has transformed into homicidal rage. When he sees his murdered children, and he kills her for it, those feelings turn into a guilt that will never leave him. He feels responsible for his children's deaths, for not giving Dolores's insanity the credence it deserved, and when he momentarily emerges from his psychotic episode, he recovers the sense of being, in fact, Andrew Laeddis, the father who wasn't there, as we shall see further on.

Gradually, we step inside the main character's unmentionable pain, and his devastating guilt. The images that walk us through his hallucinations, visions and nightmares alongside him are terrible and beautiful. Memories of the war mingle with his family tragedy, and one trauma magnifies and re-signifies the other: his seven-year-old daughter is there among the fallen war dead, her eyes open, as if asking him why he wasn't at the lake house that day to protect her and her siblings from their mother's insanity.

Daniels' "visions" translate for us the unassimilable dimensions of his pain and guilt; they are genuine nightmares. The hate, guilt, and love that he cannot transform and cannot allow to pass, along with the tragic nature of his crimes, contribute toward the impossibility of withdrawing past cathexes and investing in the present and future. Instead, he creates a neoreality, a world all of his own, to protect himself from facts too terrible to face or bear.

In this invented world, Daniels becomes a detective bent on tracking down and capturing the culprits and bringing them to justice, but his visions cannot avoid his encounter with violence and death; on the contrary, they end up compulsively replaying the sadomasochistic scene. There is nowhere Daniels can live. Neither on the island, nor off it.

His delirium makes him responsible for the entire death toll of the Second World War; he sees himself mowing down concentration camp guards, and we cannot tell if this is a memory of the war, or just another retrospective hal-lucination that expresses his real desire to murder the "guards" and doctors, the "nazis" in charge of the psychiatric hospital that has become, for him, a concentration camp. Daniels is in the grip of paranoid terror toward all figures of authority.

The reality of the facts – Dolores's madness, her killing of their kids, and his killing of her – is so terrible and full of irreconcilable emotions that the only way he can be free of the sadomasochistic scene and guilt is if he invents an avenger – Teddy Daniels – on the trail of the dangerous criminal Rachel Solando, who murdered her three children. Initially, we're caught up in the illusion, but we later discover that Rachel Solando is, in fact, a condensation of Dolores, his psychotic wife who killed their three children, and Rachel, his seven-year-old daughter who reappears in dreams and visions, staring at him in despair.

Daniels ends up confessing to his partner that he is also searching for one Andrew Laeddis, the man behind the blaze that killed his wife. Here, he refers to an earlier episode, when his wife sets fire to their apartment. Everyone was saved, but Daniels failed to detect Dolores's insanity in the arson attack on their home. In the end, we discover that Andrew Laeddis is Daniels' real name, the identity he shed because it had become uninhabitable to him. By transforming into Teddy Daniels, the avenger, he continued in search of the rejected self, which echoes back to him from reality under his actual name, as the author of his wife's murder! This is the core of truth around which his delirium is built.

At the end of the film, after briefly emerging from madness, Daniels/Laeddis regresses, and, unable to take the pain any longer, opts for lobotomy. After everything, it seems there could be no greater pain than to live on in full awareness of what transpired. The movie ends with him asking the psychiatrist the question mentioned before, whether it were really possible to go on living as a monster, knowing one is responsible for unassimilable acts.

The film has a powerful impact, deftly taking us inside madness, without knowing where we are going. Unaware that we are descending into insanity, we watch the solidity of the real collapse into delirium and hallucination.

We shall return to shared reality for a moment and look again toward our question: what makes the mourning process unfold normally and what bogs it down in the pathological mire of melancholia? We can now answer that by saying that an event of brutal violence is always hard to assimilate and allow to pass, but when it is mixed up with intense love, hate and guilt, it can form a scathingly recriminatory voice that cleaves the ego in two and erects an enclave, leaving the wounds of the past unhealed and incapable of healing. Libido then bleeds from the wound, meaning there is not enough love or forgiveness to connect and transform so many emotions. The result is the installation of an impossible mourning: melancholia.

There are four factors that contribute to the onset of melancholia and the inability to heal: the extreme tragic nature of the events, the extreme intensity of the emotions, the predominance of a Superego that is purified and unassimilable to the ego, and the patient's inability to pursue the analytic process, or to do so only intermittently, thus resulting in a negative thera-peutic reaction.

The work of Melanie Klein can help us to understand how the purified identifications of the Superego form.

Melanie Klein's contribution: purified identifications, archaic Superego, pure culture of the death drive

Why is the precocious Superego so violent? Melanie Klein believed that the originary love is voracious, devouring. In light of this sadistic love, the first parental figures are threatening, as they carry and are formed by the pro-jection of this infantile sadism, which is later re-introjected to lay the first identificatory layers of the Superego. In its origins, the Superego is sadistic and accusing – pure culture of the child's death drive projected onto the parents and re-introjected in the form of severe judgement.

The transformation of this terrifying Superego into benign moral conscience can only happen through the Ego's assimilation of much of the Superego. The sadistic aspects have to be fused with libidinal drives to create a moral and ethical conscience that involves recognition of the other and his/her rights and aspirations, and allows for the acceptance of the laws and regulations imposed by one's social community. Now, this process is nothing more or less than a mourning, which we will later call "the development of the depressive position", or, in Freudian terms, the development of the Oedipus complex.

The normal process of mourning, as described by Freud (1917), inspired Klein (1935, 1940) to devise the theory of the depressive position, a pillar of infantile development that will be responsible for the transformation of primary identifications into secondary identifications, i.e., the shift from the devouring Superego into moral and ethical conscience through mourning for the child's originary omnipotence and primitive forms of loving. This originary omnipotence is what leads the child to believe itself all-powerful, capable of doing and demanding everything it wishes, a little despot; and the process of mourning is accepting the loss of this imaginary position.

The paranoid-schizoid position, on the other hand, takes as its model the Freudian description of melancholia. Drawing upon Freud, and learning to think dialectically, Melanie Klein saw that a little melancholia is always to be found in normal mourning, and vice-versa. Both authors would agree were we to say that, in a sense, melancholia is a process of mourning that has gone awry. The dynamic aspect of Freud's thought and his idea of complementary pairs are the germs of a form of dialectical thinking that makes it impossible to approach health without also addressing illness, or illness, without the para-digm of health. Seen in this light, healing and healing-oneself are processes that aim for some far-off vanishing point while flanked all the way by possible deviations. Later, this would lead him to consider analysis an endless process (Freud, 1937). On the other hand, we might look at a successful analysis as a mourning that did not get waylaid, but contains a chain of lived episodes expanding onto new ways of living.

From the ideal good object to the good object tout court

Over the course of the depressive position, the purified ideal objects that formed the oldest layers of the Superego are gradually transformed into simple good objects; that is, neither ideal nor purely good, but good objects that emerge out of a fusing with bad ones. Another way of formulating this unification process is as follows: the good (not ideal) object needs to establish itself firmly in the ego. It is often said that a precondition of health and pre-vention of melancholia is the firm introjection of the good object. But what exactly is that? The introjection of the good object is the interiorizing, within the psychic apparatus, of the sum of one's experiences of pleasure, installing a well-established dynamic record; that is, an internal reserve of experiences of pleasure that can function as a guarantee of future access to pleasure and safety, thus boosting one's capacity to tolerate transitory experiences of pain and frustration. In this sense, the good object is more than just an archive of satisfactions, but has an efficacy and dynamism all of its own. The good object is, therefore, the name given to experiences of satisfaction that have been introjected and converted into a source of well-being and security; it's the name given to the child's experience of having its needs met in an envir-onment that can actually provide enough of what it requires. This introjected good object will be the source of the life and love instincts.

Archaic Superego and the post-Oedipal Superego: enclave and passageway

The presence of the firmly introjected good object is what makes it pos-sible for the most ferocious and savage aspects of the archaic Superego to be assimilated and metabolized, and so integrated into the ego, where they cease to function as a flashpoint of terror. The primitive Superego consists of ideal objects: the ideal positive qualities – that is, the maximum pleasure, power, and perfection – only exist by virtue of a splitting-away of ideal bad qualities (the maximum of displeasure and imperfection), which, in this ideal state, are not assimilable into the ego, and so form an obstacle, as they are impossible to translate or flesh-out symbolically. Their strictly imaginary quality leaves them static and crystalized.

But what is it that makes the strategy of purifying the good or bad quality of experiences, objects, and the subject itself so deadly? Why is it that every fundamentalist project contains a strategy to purify and destroy, and, wrapped up with that, a war plan, which, if fully executed, would end in genocide?

To purify is to separate the "good" from the "bad" in order to define a parameter for a "good" that permits no imperfection. This "good" has to be "pure". Once the bad has been isolated away, it can then be eradicated and destroyed; it's a procedure that corresponds to the omnipotent fantasy of sloughing off every stain, defect, or sub-par trait in order to become entirely good.

The delirious reason behind fundamentalisms is created out of this belief in pure ideals; and the projection of "badness" upon "others", whether people or peoples (Bruneteau, 2005; Semelin, 2009; Cintra, 2001).

The idea of a pure good and bad incites condemning judgements and the projection of these ideals, creating idols and scapegoats. A judgement based on moral certainties, which withholds benefit of the doubt and shuts down any weighing of viewpoints, necessarily leads to a "final solution" and death. This kind of delirious reason casts its shadow on the "other", which it is fated to eliminate, because it represents a threat by virtue of being different to the I – and so intrinsically "bad".

Purifying and destroying are, therefore, extreme defensive strategies that aim to deal with paranoid angst, and the threat which the other, the different to the I, represents: the other is now branded a dangerous enemy that is poised to attack. The I must pre-empt that attack, characterize the other's "badness" categorically, grounded solely on difference to self, then destroy it at all costs, before it can destroy the I. It's the modus operandi of the archaic Superego and its primary identifications; an "all or nothing" regime of "final solutions".

When mourning is possible, we see that the Superego mellows, and primary identifications soften into secondary identifications, developed at length during the depressive position; in fact, during various depressive positions, or, in Freudian terms, through the development of the Oedipus and castration complexes.

On the side of illness, what remains is the cleaving apart of the ego, and the formation of an enclave impervious to movement and the passage of time. Repetition takes hold, along with a rejection and lack of creative work. We might consider this the work of the death drive, or the work of melancholia, set against symbolization and the passage of time.

On the side of health, we have the work of dream and mourning, the symbolization of lack and absence, access to play, transitionality and the capacity to love, care, and work. Temporalization is only possible through a well-developed mourning process. On this side, we find what André Green calls the "work of the negative" (Green, 1993, 1999).

Winnicott's contribution to the conditions that favor mourning: from devastating guilt to the capacity for concern and responsibility

In "The Development of the Capacity for Concern", Winnicott (1963) developed his theory that the devastating feeling of guilt that arises in the first depressive positions needs to transform into the capacity for concern, responsibility-taking, and commitment to people and tasks. In melancholia, the guilt is so crushing that it has to be expelled and rejected. When the feeling of guilt cannot be felt and processed, but needs to be violently denied, the path is lain for the most gratuitous and arbitrary acts of violence. Freud (1916) had foreseen as much when he wrote about criminals who committed crimes when overcome by a terrible guilt. On the other hand, Winnicott is thinking about situations of health, when the mourning of the depressive position can unfurl and the feeling of guilt can indeed emerge, be contained, and finally be transformed through the maturational process. Speaking of the conversion of guilt into concern, the author writes:

> The word 'concern' is used to cover in a positive way a phenomenon that is covered in a negative way by the word 'guilt'. A sense of guilt is anxiety linked with the concept of ambivalence, and implies a degree of integration in the individual ego that allows for the retention of good object-imago along with the idea of a destruction of it. Concern implies further integration, and further growth, and relates in a positive way to the individual's sense of responsibility, especially in respect of relationships into which the instinctual drives have entered. Concern refers to the fact that the individual cares, or minds, and both feels and accepts responsibility.
>
> (Winnicott, 1963/1983, p. 73)

Winnicott thinks that an ability to show concern for the other lies at the root of all play, work, and creative endeavor. However, this transformation of the feeling of guilt into concern can only happen if the environment is favorable. The transformation occurs during the stage in which the baby can combine aggressive and erotic impulses, that is, when it attains ambivalence. The refinement of ambivalence is what will give rise to the capacity for concern.

He also reasons that the Id-drives that generate the various libidinal phases (oral, anal, urethral, phallic) are connected to fantasies of attack and destruction, of devouring and taking possession of the maternal body. The fantasy is experienced as if it were real, and if the mother survives these attacks, the child takes this as being due to her survival capacity, and will feel extremely grateful. When all this can occur, the conditions are favorable. The child feels guilt over the Id-drives, but also sees that the mother has survived its attacks and that it can perhaps make amends through play, communication, and a calmer form of relating. This set of circumstances gives the baby the chance to make reparations, shifting from primitive guilt to the ability to care and accept responsibility.

Winnicott's main contribution is the idea that the good enough environment and maternal presence – and that of the analyst capable of being there to receive the spontaneous gesture after the attacks of primitive love – are decisive factors in making mourning possible and avoiding the deviations of course that lead to melancholia and other psychotic states. However, sometimes circumstances prevail in which no environment seems good enough to receive these gestures of reparation, and in which not all gestures of reparation seem good enough to enable the child to accept the traumatic reality.

The only way out in such a situation is to close oneself away in delirium and deny the reality of the facts.

The analytical process is the installation of a good enough environment that offers a way out of this omnipotent state through the process of mourning. Some psychotics and fundamentalists never mourn this omnipotence, which implies learning to live with one's own imperfections and those of others, and with the sense of groundlessness, transitoriness, loss and death. Analysis could provide this opportune window of time during which the patient could be accompanied in the courageous gesture of wading into the river of trans-formations, letting go of the past, of self-torture and violence. But it is very difficult to give up magical thinking when the reality of the facts is as devas-tating as the one facing the main character of *Shutter Island*.

The analyst's ethics demands that he remains at hand, even if the vio-lence of reality renders all his devices and offerings insufficient. It is in this limitrophe that the analysand's capacity to feel and think is put to the test, as are the chances of his experiencing mourning. The entire personal analysis is strength-tested, and often nothing, or very little, can be done for the other. It's an immersion in the other's darkness, a sloughing-off of certainties, a time to call everything into doubt, and begin to learn again from scratch.

The Third Bank of the River[6]

> In this third millennium, he ordered the murder of American women because they do not cover their faces, because they smoke, drink, con-verse with men as equals, and, the supreme boldness of it, choose their own sexual partners, refusing to submit to marriages arranged for them by the clan. If anyone thinks I am exaggerating here, take a look at the manifestos circulating online denouncing the abuse of Afghan women...
> José Nêumane (O Estado De São Paulo, 10/10/2001, p. A2)

The terrorist attacks that took place in the United States on September 11, 2001, made me think that the most important task in combating the spread of hatred on a global scale would be a persistent and in-depth exercise in thinking capable of exposing and debunking the logic that underpins fun-damentalism and terrorist practices. I liken this effort to the millennia-long process of water eroding stone: the harder the rock, the more surprising is the water's insidious power to eat away at it and dissolve it. I think of the fertile earth with its groundwaters, the vast phreatic reserves that ensure the mir-acle of germination. I think of certain priceless moments of contact with the other and the other's alterity. I was lost in daydreams as I prepared to write this text, and then a person very dear to me came out with the expression "água da palavra" (the water of words), from the Caetano Veloso song "A Terceira Margem do Rio" (The Third Bank of the River). "But isn't that a story by Guimarães Rosa, from the book Primeiras Estórias? – I asked. Yes, exactly.

Veloso composed the song while reflecting on Rosa's tale about a father who decides to withdraw from all contact with his family by rowing out to an invisible horizon: the third bank of the river. But what third bank is this? Where is it? Is it half-way across? Is it a transitional space, a space of possibilities? Removing himself from all the chatter, from the positivity of presence, where did this father actually go? Did he absence himself in order to make way for the other, for their alterity? Questions that await an answer. For the time being, here are some of Caetano's verses: Água da palavra, água calada pura. Água da palavra, água de rosa dura. Proa da palavra, duro silêncio, nosso pai. Margem da palavra. Entre as escuras duas Margens da palavra Clareira, luz madura Rosa da palavra Puro silêncio, nosso pai. (The water of words, purest silent water. Water of words, water from the hardest rose. The water's prow, hard silence, our father. The word's shores. Between the two dark banks of the word. Clearing, mature light. Rose of the word. Pure silence, our father).

I am extremely grateful to the person who presented me this poetic horizon toward which to reflect on hate and intolerance. From that very moment, I felt, as I wrote, that persuasive, refreshing power flowing behind the letters and thoughts. Water of words. Mysterious power to slake thirst and make thoughts sprout. I had found the third bank, and the water ran from this encounter with the other.

The other encounter

I arrived at the consultancy, as on so many other Fridays before, but this time it was a friend, not a patient, who had come to talk. I began to listen to him, his pain, his slow rhythm, full of pauses, his words escaping from the stone throat, from the unpronounceable claw that keeps us isolated from one another. Some words began to spatter like raindrops on the floor, tapping out the sounds of "other-ness", "alter-ity", pitter-pattering on the stone like anti-missiles of peace, resounding, echoing. I started listening attentively to the delicious, fragile music tenderizing the floor beneath our feet, and making it warp into the background. I felt myself melting inside, without yet understanding what it all meant, but being able to sense in the man the dissolution of old certainties and some solitary, childhood pains. My unsatisfied hungers gave way, as did all feelings of humiliation and the oppression of need; in short, everything that had the power to turn me into a potential terrorist just fell away. Resentment caved under the weight of all that water and I was deliciously incapable of holding it back. That man's words were like deep, nutrient-rich waters that made reserves of emotion, thousands of years old, suddenly flourish: I was simply the site of that mysterious happening. How can words have so much power? A silent tilth, furrow, mark, the water of words, word-breeze. And it had enough force to tear down one world and build another in its place.

I had embarked on the voyage of listening to him, though I still did not know where it was leading, but the pain expressed was accompanied by a deep sense of gratitude. Over the course of this journey through his pain, he completed a new crossing and gifted me the possibility of contact with those hidden reserves of unshed tears. I understood why it was so difficult to experience loss and to cry for what we mourn, and why we fling ourselves into our little daily acts of terrorism. Flight from words. Violence thrives when we cannot tap into the wells of suppressed tears and the dark, dizzying resentment, which no words could ever express. I felt that I needed to prepare a deeper reservoir of silence and celebrate my own mournings more thoroughly. I had to bury the dead I had distractedly left strewn about the landscapes of my life. If I failed to complete that work of words, if I did not tend to it as a matter of urgency, I would be making my own personal contribution to the world's violence.

Elucidating violence itself is only part of a greater effort to understand the violence infiltrating the fundamentalist logic that informs acts of terror. The question is wide-ranging, and requires that we gather together everything that has been thought to date about the inexhaustible violence of humankind and our difficulty in dealing with the other, without immediately wanting to assimilate or devour that other into our own beliefs and values.

Melanie Klein helps to elucidate violence

The psychoanalyst Melanie Klein systematically studied the question of aggressiveness and hatred, and her thinking can make a valuable contribution to its elucidation. After all the destruction and death of that September Tuesday, I remember a friend telling me that I could safely tell my students that Melanie Klein had good reasons for building her theory around the phenomenon of hatred and destructiveness smoldering tirelessly in hearts and minds. In these sombre times of terror and fundamentalism, the emphasis she placed on destructiveness and aggressiveness frames it as a key point, one that had drawn Freud's interest since the First World War, with his studies of obsessive neurosis and melancholia. Freud was deeply impressed by the presence of masochism, sadism, aggressiveness, and hatred, which could hardly be derived from the libido alone. In addition to the infinite and rapacious desire for love (Sehnsucht), which Freud postulated, and perhaps even as a result of the impossibility of satisfying this insatiable demand, the conditions are created for the emergence of all forms of violence.

Some of these have their origins in the environment: the violence of misery that cuts off the circulation of goods people need to live, the result of a vitiated system for the distribution of wealth; and the violence of ideological and religious systems, which establish and define the modes of circulation, at the same time as they create a value system and impediments that foster exclusion and fanatical radicalization. On the psychic side, the sheer power of drive-based demands, the violence of the imaginary and interiorized prohibitions are capable of reproducing and amplifying, ad infinitum, the violence of ideology and religion.

Archaic angsts

For Melanie Klein, psychic violence pre-dates the capacity to love; it comes before the ability to think, postpone, act, or generate resources and projects. Before everything else, we are this: a sheaf of violent needs and demands, mired in the most afflictive groundlessness. In other words, before we begin to perceive and desire the other as an other, with capacity to keep our distance and stand in difference to that other, we are pure vampiric, voracious need – a whirlwind of archaic angsts and desires that make us indiscernible from others; we are hosts of the purest violence of the imaginary, and that leaves us helpless. The violence of this hankering to incorporate and possess the other and the voracity that characterizes the most primitive form of love make for a dangerous and threatening world, generated through projection, because the world we encounter out there is impregnated with this incorporative yearning. That's where these persecutory archaic angsts come from. But what does Klein mean to say by this?

Persecutory angsts are so called because they foster the sensation that we are being persecuted and attacked. They are terrors, like the nameless terrors of falling without end, of having our Ego annihilated, or of being abandoned, killed, invaded, devoured, or destroyed by a monstrous power against which we have no defense. The image of being swallowed by a huge wave or snatched by a shark or other "monster" can all be figurations of the most archaic persecutory angsts.

Primitive defenses

Set against the violence of drives and the imaginary, it becomes essential that we create defense mechanisms that can, in a sense, abate and appease the intensity of these first angsts. One of those mechanisms is splitting, which consists in radically cleaving good experiences (those that generate pleasure) from the bad (those that engender any form of displeasure, discomfort, or pain).

Melanie Klein believes that experiences of pleasure are attributed to a person, the mother, who then becomes the good mother, the provider of care and love. On the other hand, bad experiences are attributed to the mother who frustrates, punishes, or leaves the child's needs unmet. In other words, in earliest life, psychism organizes its experiences into those that cause pleasure and displeasure, polarizing both and holding one up as the ideally good object and the other as a terrible persecutor.

The dynamism that separates the purified good from the radical bad is present in the logic of fundamentalism, which preaches the absolute goodness of God versus the evil of the infidels, who must be annihilated for their sins. Formulating an absolute, unattainable "good" preserves it from all contamination, so it can be eternalized in its incorruptibility: it becomes an imaginary reserve of "the good" that can last forever, which is exactly what we most deeply desire.

On the other hand, the major advantage of standing in opposition to an object that is absolutely bad is that there is no doubt about what needs to be done with it: the persecutor must be destroyed; mercilessly annihilated. Formulating an object as fully evil, I can justify any act of violence against it. If I am vanquishing it in the name of the Supreme Good, then the end justifies any means, because they will be "holy" and "blessed": the bearer of my projection of pure evil is stripped of all subjectivity, right to defense, and rights per se; it is disposability incarnate, mere dejecta.

However, in order to create an ideally good object, I must deny any lack or flaw it might contain; that's part of the idealization necessary if the immaculately good and perfect object – a veritable God – is to arise.

Melanie Klein considered denial a powerful archaic defense mechanism designed to annihilate any undesirable aspects in people. As such, it is intimately tied to idealization. Those who manage to approximate to this extreme quality of the Good – martyrs, saints, and priests – are closer to God (or Alah, for Muslims). Therein resides the danger of fanaticism. If God is inaccessible in his metaphorical realm of the absolute goodness, we can never really know what his will might be. The danger lies in judging our mullahs or priests sufficiently legitimate representatives and spokespersons for the Absolute Good that they will able to translate it for us: that is what leads to a regressive shift that blindly submits us to God's will, just as one day in the past we were obliged to obey our parents. From that moment on, all manner of arbitrary action can be committed in the name of the Supreme God, whose will has been passed down to us through his oracles and chosen-ones.

The discovery of the diary kept by one of the terrorists who organized the American attacks reveals his profound conviction: by killing and destroying Americans, the representatives of Satan, he would be doing the will of the Supreme God. This fanatic discourse betrays the absolute certainty that characterizes psychotic states: there was no doubt whatsoever that the Americans were satanists and that the plan to kill them was a gesture of obedience to the Supreme Good. There was no room for doubt, questioning, criticism, meditation, or reflection. Through Jihad (which means blind obedience to God's will), Taliban fundamentalism transforms words and beliefs into warheads to be launched against the other; that is, against all those who do not share the same beliefs and values and have therefore been duly "satanized".

There is another defense mechanism for dealing with the emotional turbulence of early life which Melanie Klein describes, and that's flight to the good object, which consists in imaginarily seeking refuge at the "heart of the ideal good object", which allows us to deny our own fragility and groundlessness and to embark on the delicious adventure of sharing in divine omnipotence. The most seductive promise of fundamentalism is the chance to become powerful, indeed omnipotent, which can be considered a strategy for recovering power and triumphing over the frailty of human existence.

We can admit that the feeling of omnipotence in early life is an important defense: the child denies its fragility, impotence and helplessness in those earliest times. The more defenseless and immature the child, the greater the sense of omnipotence and of being the center of the universe will be.

Melanie Klein showed that psychic development consists in the painful process of losing this sense of omnipotence and centrality: it entails relinquishing the throne of "his majesty, the baby". The principle of reality demands that we all confront ourselves with our own ignorance, impotence, and the demands of necessity, which establish different degrees of dependence and learning. Now, in order to accept that I am a creature of necessity, subject to sickness and death, incapable of satisfying the majority of my needs alone, I necessarily have to abdicate this sense of omnipotence and self-sufficiency. This painful mourning process makes me cry and lament, at the same time as I continue nourishing the most secret desire to reclaim that power and triumph over vulnerability. Feeling the center of attentions and indeed the world was so pleasureful, while having to endure a mediocre humdrum or even miserable life is intolerable and tedious by comparison with those grandiose earliest experiences of power and plenitude! Therein lies the fertile ground for religious fanaticism and fundamentalism.

The more intense the desire to reclaim lost omnipotence and the deeper the disdain for the meagre acquisitions of everyday life, the more susceptible one becomes to the allure of all forms of nazism and fascism. These ideologies promise to restore our originary perfection and omnipotence through association with some Almighty figure and his representatives on earth.

Suicide as the promise of restored plenitude

However, if we cling to this growing and increasingly voracious aspiration to recover our early state of omnipotence and plenitude, we run the risk of going into a tailspin that culminates in melancholic-type suicide. Many psychoanalytic authors have written about this boundary experience. Killing oneself, in this case, means destroying the precarious nature of a body and an existence that are now lived in the key of lack, vulnerability and insufficiency. It's an asphyxiating logic that produces an insidious, silent transformation of the body and one's own existence into waste to be discarded. This downward spiral starts with countless lighter forms of maligning life – labeled frustrating, precarious, flawed – and of demeaning the self – branded unworthy, insufferable – until it finally sinks to the nadir of codifying this real living body under its most extreme classification yet: as fecal matter. It's a reduction that makes suicide a glorious act, a fast-track to reclaimed grandiosity.

Death is not sought as an end in itself, as the extinguishing of life, but as a gateway to true fullness, the cessation of all the conflict, need and pain of existence: committing suicide becomes a strategy for recovering the most absolute narcissistic plenitude. Opting for death is not so hard when life has been devalued to such an extent that it is no better than fecal matter. The body and life have been utterly reified, so it is no longer difficult to view them as a price worth paying for the greater good. In this we see the grandiose sensation of being in the service of a heroic mission of purification that will eradicate evil. The splendor of the mission eclipses the insignificance of existence; giving up this meaningless life in exchange for eternal life beyond it seems a small price to pay. Suicide is carried out not to destroy oneself, but to remake the originary immaculateness of existence.

In this sort of death we see the search for a supreme and monumental meaning that can fill the emptiness of life. It's the most extreme act of omnipotence and the refusal to accept the anonymous human condition. It represents triumph over the impotence, triviality, and precariousness of a humdrum existence rife with misery and insignificance.

Shedding infantile omnipotence: the depressive position

For Melanie Klein, emerging from the most chronic state of omnipotence is a long, drawn-out process of mourning that begins at birth and continues through to death. It is true that psychotics, some highly narcissistic or schizoid personalities and fanatics of sects in general never go through the transformation process which the author calls "the depressive position" (note that here "depressive" does not refer to the psychopathological condition of depression).

An aspect of this transformation can be illustrated with a political metaphor. The Cold War revealed a stark political division between the United States, on one side, and the Soviet Union, on the other, which allowed the globe to be divided schematically into right and left. Since the fall of the Berlin Wall, however, and the collapse of the USSR and of the Russian plan to globalize the communist revolution, the political panorama has become more complex and difficult than before. Such was the confusion engendered by this new ambivalent geopolitical panorama that the world crept back into its old modus of "we, the good" versus "them, the bad". In other words, there was a deeper regression to isolated acts of fanatical destruction best described as cries of despair or uncoordinated, anarchic movements. Something analogous happens when we slip into the depressive position. In the earlier phase (paranoid-schizoid), a clear line could be drawn between the good and the bad, and those considered "bad" could be annihilated as dangerous persecutors. Unpleasant, uncomfortable experiences were jettisoned and evacuated, or projected onto the world and upon "others".

In the depressive position, however, we begin to see a confluence between love and hate: objects are no longer viewed as exclusively good or bad, the belief that the world is populated by heroes and villains is shed, and the positive and negative characteristics attributed to oneself and to others are relativized. A new panorama emerges that reveals a more complex psychic reality. There is growing recognition of one's own aggression, which makes it difficult to sustain the belief that all the "badness" is in the world or in the "other".

The psychic reality begins to display enhanced tension due to the presence of conflict that gives rise to guilt, remorse, and a desire for reparation. We experience tremendous disappointment, because the ideal, perfect, absolutely giving object ceases to exist. The child begins to realize that the mother that feeds is also the mother that frustrates, and that nobody is infallible and inexhaustible; there is a very disturbing shift in the quality of the good object. The perfect, omnipresent mother is replaced with one that functions "well enough", but which can also fail and cause anguish. A new parental image emerges that is tainted with imperfection and damaged in its completeness. This causes sorrow and an afflicted sense of responsibility toward others. The need to be tended to and cared for is reduced and there is a nascent desire to care for and protect the other. The child develops a higher tolerance threshold in relation to other people's failings.

This position is called "depressive" because it involves a process of mourning, which consists in accepting the loss of the ideal aspects of people and the development of a capacity to let go of our more radical representations that demand "everything, absolutely good". Instead, we accept and instal new representations of "something, relatively good". The magnificent child dies, and a new subjectivity begins to form. It is a shift from the "splendid cradle" of the Brazilian national anthem to a new bearing that accepts responsibility.

However, the move into the depressive position is the hardest transformation of all, and entails every imaginable type of regression to the prior position. It's not easy to abdicate the status of the magnificent infant and step into the regime of reality, which demands that we postpone the satisfaction of our needs, turn to work, recognize the other in their difference and develop the capacity to think, feel, and tolerate frustration. Heaped upon the anxieties that haunt our earliest life are those that come with the depressive position, and our problems become infinitely more complex: this gives rise to a strong regressive shift back towards the paranoid-schizoid position, which is very recognizable in maniacal defenses. These defenses speak to the difficulty the subject is having in entering the process of mourning this lost omnipotence; they are tendencies to try to reclaim the lost status and return to a simpler, more dualistic organization of the world.

Mechanisms to defend the paranoid-schizoid position involve radical schisms between the Absolute Good and Radical Bad and strategies to evacuate and destroy everything that causes discomfort. In the depressive position, on the other hand, the child looks for new ways of working through the psychic chaos and drive-based violence. These new methods are more introjective: the child develops greater tolerance of the discomfort that comes with being bombarded by contradictory drives and acquires enhanced capacity to bear conflict between different aspects of experience. All of this is to say that heavier psychic work and greater capacity to delay gratification become essential. The result is that, at the end of this painstaking labor of shouldering responsibility for events, we are better equipped to make use of impulse energy and integrate it into the Ego.

The mechanisms of the depressive position can be compared with a slow gestation, because it involves the creation of new potential space or psychic "space" in which pictorial and verbal representation will be worked on and modified, avoiding wholesale discharge of instinctive energies through actions.

The metaphor of psychic "space" is always unreliable, as it segues directly into visuality, into images and the imaginary, with its violent strategies to capture and crystallize thought. Perhaps we might think of a virtual space instead, a place that is hidden and invisible, a non-topos or "no place" where we can be relatively free from the capture and prison of the imaginary. To understand this shift from the idealized imagos of infancy to relative solitude and full capacity to think that comes with maturity – through the depressive position – we might look to the story "The Third Bank of the River".

Entering this position is not easy; but crossing through it is even harder: if the riverbanks are absolute beliefs, we must leave them, sail free of them, head towards the middle of the river. The depressive position demands that we let gods and demons die and abandon our childhood beliefs that there is a good and a bad that can be clearly separated off in their purified states. There can only be true growth when our idols fall and disappear along with the idea of a magical, immediatist thinking. This latter mindset needs to be replaced with a genuine exercise in pondering over, feeling, and working through conflicts, and the development of the ability to coexist with what is alien to us, whilst tolerating pain and frustration and accepting the human condition of groundlessness, transitoriness, and finitude. These are tasks for a lifetime, which is why they say we never bring the depressive position to completion. It is a deep dive into the other's darkness, into a life shorn of certainties and awash with doubt.

The Third Bank of the River: a place of possibilities

The third bank of the river is the place of words, the water of words. It is the house of words. Where silence dwells. In Guimarães Rosa's story, a father retreats to this place beyond the reach of the familiar, an enigmatic place, a non-existent third bank of the river. What does that mean? It means the father has withdrawn into an inaccessible, ungraspable place; he does not want to be trapped in any schema or code. He will not allow for totalizing understanding.

Judaic tradition speaks of the unpronounceability of God's name. Inability to say his name corresponds to the "no place" of the third bank; it is the "father's" insistence on remaining inaccessible to our all-petrifying imaginary, off in some other dimension. This embargo on "imaginizing" God is an important limit to the insatiable activity of the imaginary and language, a way of imposing silence on the banks of the word: in a sense, God sheds his substantiveness to become a verb.

As a verb, "father" is the bestowal of life. Some would say the signifier father is this generative capacity, this engendering, begetting, being capable of such authorship: father is a vital principle. But we must think of parenthood metaphorically, as the capacity to bear fruit, to fructify. Think of fatherhood, that is, in terms of pure activity, the activity of giving being: from the static image to the movement that suggests instantaneity, presentness, always re-beginning; an incessant gushing of water from the spring.

And so the spatial metaphor of gestation as a "psychic space" begins to temporalize: the father is now the activity of being and of bestowing being, of bringing to be, and letting be. To let the other be we must step away, cancel ourselves, stand by, row out to the third bank of the river, become "absently present". Many of those to whom I told Rosa's story were incensed by the father's indifference, adrift in the middle of the river like that. But is it indifference or the opening of space, a genuine bearing toward the other? A certain indifference, a little discontinuity is necessary to fatherhood, so that the child can fully emerge: being a father is to say après vous, mes enfants.

Third bank and third party

I see these as lessons learned from Levinas (1971), in Totality and Infinity, when he suggests that we should allow the idea of the infinite to dissolve the totalitarianism of the imaginary. This father who refuses to phenomenalize and absconds to the invisible, is a principle of infinity that has come to shatter any desire for omnipotence, any aspiration towards perfection, and all the totalitarianism of the ego.

The infinite is that which is still pending, it is the principle of incomplete-ness. And as incomplete, it is yet to come; is always becoming anew. This father, as invisible alterity, relativizes, decentralizes and destabilizes the I in its despotic position, immersed in its illusion of self-sufficiency.

Being "totally other", pure difference, the desire to stand apart, this father is, himself, the third margin that overflows the narcissistic immersions of the I in the you and the you in the I. He is alterity that breaks from the sameness installed by the specular and seductive "face to face" of the scopic drive; the third margin that relativizes fascination, the sideration of the Great Other.

Rather than presence himself, the father that goes to the third bank of the river dissolves into the unseen, out there on the horizon of possibilities, in the shapeless void. This recalls Levinas' notion of the "Third party" (1971), that "illeity" that is the ungraspable, ever-enigmatic dimension in the other and in oneself. Without the "illeity" of oneself and the other, that indissoluble core of alterity, nothing could escape the assimilative voracity of the ego.

The enigmatic father of the third bank of the river is the foreign, the surplus of meaning, which the I cannot assimilate: it is, above all, the silence that sets questioning, doubt and uncertainty in motion. Striking out to this invisible bank, the father experiences a way "otherwise than being", of withdrawing, so that the other can be. The third bank is that place propitious to the giving of being.

Pure silence, our father. Considering the effects of terrorist fanaticism, I ask myself: If the fundamentalist God, in his triumphant majesty and most obscene monstrousness, can incite so much bloodshed, what do we still need the Devil for? Surely this God Almighty would be quite enough, stained as he is with blood, obscenity, and the lust for destruction, forever demanding the most radical passiveness and utter obedience (jihad) to his will. The final act of all fundamentalism is suicide, because the dynamism of this God leads to death: the insidious strategy of injecting hate and disdain into the body and into life is the very call to disembody.

On the other hand, the figuration of this silent father on the third bank of the river serves as a counterweight to the most archaic and totalitarian paternal imagoes that oppress with the crushing weight of their shadows. Pure silence, our father. To counterbalance this triumphant, bloodthirsty God, we need to find the third bank of the river, a horizon where we can shed our passional, murderous certainty and need to be an omnipresent everything.

Melanie Klein would say that, as we work through the depressive position, we re-manage all our idols: the all-powerful mother and father and the magnificent, despotic child. There is a loss of glow and grandiosity, but gains in terms of consideration for others, for those beyond myself. That makes me think that what these fundamentalists need is to allow their bloodthirsty, narcissistic almighty god to die so they can find their own way to the third bank of the river and to the silence of the Father. In the midst of the father, we must discern the son. The God of the 21st Century is a fragile, helpless child crying with hunger and thirst; in need of the water of words. He has entrusted the adults with the task of pacifying the world. No appeal. "Time for words, When nothing is said, beyond words. When the innermost blooms. Wings of the word, wings now folded in. House of the word, where silence dwells. Pure silence, our father."

On the feeling of solitude[7]

After all, might it not be a case for the patient to come to analysis so as to reconstruct his solitude through the other; the solitude that he alone can know?

The patient comes to analysis in order to experience this intriguing solitude "à deux" in order to reconstruct a world that only he can know. It's a case of restoring the capacity to be alone in someone else's company so as to make contact with oneself and the other without succumbing to the temptation to "become one and the same" with that other. Such an adventure requires that we enter into a non-instrumental, non-focused state in which we are receptive to present and past memories and desires, but without fixating on any of them. The goal is to float through sensorial psychic reality toward that place Bion spoke of where there is "neither memory nor desire"; a remote place where dreams and psychic life are generated. Along the way, we must create a transitional space, a playground in which mutual engagement will turn up nexuses and connections between present sensations and past stimuli, elements of dream and of vigil, within and without, self and other.

In "The Capacity to Be Alone" (1958), Winnicott evokes these moments of contact and silence, which a patient can experience in analysis. They are, perhaps, the only times in our lives when we succeed in being truly alone without feeling isolated or shut inside ourselves. These are moments marked by a pleasant feeling of intimacy, a capacity to occupy oneself with one's own things, one's own world of inner objects, all the stuff that is capable of absorbing and enthralling us most deeply. A child lost in play is perhaps the first manifestation of this phenomenon. If today we were to ask Winnicott if he considered the capacity to be alone one of the criteria for the end of analysis, he would certainly say "yes", because something so apparently humdrum actually demands a considerable level of autonomy and consolidated sense of the self and other, which only comes from a deep reserve of well-developed primary maternal experience.

This was the road Winnicott took: he looked into the roots of this capacity, and the conditions that enable it. The capacity to be alone is grounded in the earliest relationship with the mother – and herein lies a paradox: being alone demands the presence and relaxed company of someone else, by your side, absently available, someone with whom you can have contact at any time, whether in outer reality or in the virtual reality of your inner world.

When the interior world seems to be made up of living beings, voices from the past and the present that mix and meld in relative harmony, forming a space of conviviality that seems more like a cosmos than a chaos, it is precisely then – or rather, out of that relatively ordered and vital inner world – that we acquire the capacity to be alone in someone else's presence.[8]

Perhaps the first solitude we feel in childhood is that of inhabiting a body and a history in a unique and non-transferrable way. At the same time, we learn to speak and communicate with others who appear to understand us, at least most of the time, and we develop some level of intimacy with our bodies and with our loves, hates, suspicions, certainties, guilts, and absolutions. But there are times when we find ourselves immersed in a profound sense of incommunicability, in which words are useless; generating more noise than understanding.

The analytical encounter invites the patient to lie down on the divan, bracket out her habitual rules of social interaction, and abandon herself to the free-flow of associations, gazing away toward this haze of unpredictability, while allowing her words to take her on a trip – or roller-coaster ride – in space and time. The divan becomes a magic carpet, or flying bed, like the ones in Frida Kahlo's paintings. It's an invitation to become something like the flâneur who wanders about the unknown city, freed from the commute between home and a routine destination. Like the flâneur, we saunter down back-alleys and side streets.

In the meantime, the analyst sits in silence and at hand, always a foot or two behind, remembering that a lot of what is being said is history and that the analysand has to let the past be the past. She invites the patient to release his certainties, his load-bearing truths. She is always rather incredulous, with that blank expression, silently listening and occasionally asking "Really, though?", inserting tiny wedges of doubt into those rock-solid beliefs. She is unmoving, but her motor-sensory immobility is the very effort in itself to transform all the turbulence of her own psychic life into a state of listening and openness. I like to think of the analyst as wanting to become, herself, a grounding openness. She latches onto what is most unsettled – the other's flow and dynamism – without failing to accompany her own fluctuating rhythm.

In addition to Winnicott, the analyst Christopher Bollas (1999) said: "each encounter with a patient sends me deeply into myself, to a place of essential solitude ruled by inaudible laws of dense mental complexity".

In the analytical session, the very fact that we are alone there, in the plural, reveals an invisible community, a being-alone in good company. All of this begins with the quality of a maternal presence capable of creating an environment of trust and safety, which gives the child the freedom to play, invent, and express him/herself bodily and verbally, and which is held in reserve going forward, unintrusively, in calm silence, creating what we referred to as a potential space. It is, therefore, a state of solitude devoid of abandonment or isolation.

Winnicott tells us that, very often, finding ourselves faced with a difficult problem, we withdraw into an inner space, which he calls "my club", a place of intimacy and interlocution. For an Englishman, the idea of belonging to a peer club is the realization of an ideal of harmonious, fruitful conviviality, which this analyst so frequently practiced. Filling oneself with trusted human presences in such a friendly "atmosphere" requires the negation of full presences, which can be invasive and loud. The intuition of the negative[9], an element present in Winnicott's thought and further developed by André Green, affirms the possibility that reality, in its sensorial fullness, allows itself to be negated and forgotten; only then can it become psychic reality. We might say that allowing oneself to be negated and interiorizing oneself are two different ways of speaking of the same phenomenon. Only human presence capable of disappearing without becoming entirely absent can become voice, name, figure, and memory assimilated by the nascent subject as the bricks-and-mortar of its new subjectivity.

Our destiny is to interiorize meaningful experiences: "Our life passes in change. And ever-shrinking the outer diminishes" (Rilke, 1922). The forward march of life forces us to replace that "outer" with living internal objects, integrated and humanized. These are, mainly, moments of maternal care, when we were fed and cuddled, and of the paternal function of separating and discriminating what will have to become absently available, so that we can live in peace and become our own person. The simple act of going to sleep, of letting ourselves doze off – wrapped in the arms of Morpheus, since the times of Greek mythology – is only possible in the visible or invisible arms of someone who can imitate the comfortable lap of those earliest times. And not only falling asleep; waking also requires the other's embrace. Without it, how could we rise and face the overbearing reality of this world day after day? Once again we're presented with the paradox that being alone requires the real or interiorized presence of someone capable of holding us, caring for us, and listening to us.

But living with others also demands the capacity to be alone. Someone told me of their intense need to be by their girlfriend's side in a state of calm indifference, and how hard it was for her to understand that desire. So he made an extreme yet simple appeal: "pretend I'm a dog, I'll talk to you when I can". It's a request to be left aside, playing alone, entertained by his own thoughts, and of having his full presence, in a sense, denied, yet without ever being completely absent. It's not a masochistic appeal to be mistreated – in the common sense of "treated like a dog" –, just left alone in his purest animality, immersed in a pre-verbal existence. What's more, it's an invitation for his girlfriend to join him in this calm state of indifference to every explicit manifestation of love or consideration. The other has to be able to handle the feeling of being excluded from part of the other's psychic life, leaving him to a world of inner objects that are unknown to her, and should remain so. It also entails feeling free to exclude the other, without succumbing to the unhealthy guilt that demands participation and sharing.

In a short poem titled "Casamento" (Marriage)[10], Adélia Prado (1971) describes a couple who, after years of living together, find themselves in just this state of silent, implicit communion:

> There are women who say:
> Husband, if you want to fish, go fish,
> but see that you clean the catch.
> Not I. Whatever the hour, night or day, I rise
> And help descale them, dice them, salt them up.
> It's so nice just the two of us in the kitchen,
> Every now and then our elbows brush,
> And he'll say "this one fought hard".
> "Drew silver circles in the air, slapping its tail".
> And he'll make the gesture with his hand.
> The silence of the first time we saw each other
> Runs through the kitchen, deep as a river.
> And finally, with the fish on a platter,
> We head off to bed.
> Silvery things sizzle:
> We are bride and groom.

In fact, the capacity to be alone in someone else's presence rekindles the enigma of relationships between people and the way each has laid his or her own path toward the other, this "fellow" (nebenmensch, in Freud), at once so familiar and so foreign… How much proximity and how much distance does there have to be between myself and the other for there to exist love and intimacy, recognition and authorization, even if always encircled by the risk of over-dependence or domination? Moreover, how are we to build an inner world that makes it possible to recognize others without being threatened, undermined, subjugated, violated, invaded, or ignored by them? How can we resist the desire to control or possess the other?

A peaceful human environment and parents who could grant and accept authorizations favor the interiorization of feminine and masculine figures that stand apart from each other whilst maintaining mutual contact. It keeps tension to a minimum that allows for union and, at the same time, separation; as such, each pole – the masculine and the feminine – can coexist without canceling the other out. On the other hand, an atmosphere of disdain, rivalry, aggression, and abandonment will favor the interiorization of a chaotic world in which the characters attack or demean each other; and under these conditions it is very common for the masculine to become despotic and authoritarian, behaving towards the feminine in the key of contempt (or viceversa). The figures of men and women combine in sadomasochistic[11] form, creating the combined-parent figure, in which there is neither differentiation nor union.[12]

These primitive fantasies are experienced by every new child that comes into the world and they express the child's sexual life and destructiveness; they are gradually forged in a unique combination that gathers together the influences of the environment and the reactions of each individual to a world of significant life events. Becoming a new subject requires becoming the heir to everything which this environment has to offer, including the unsavory aspects of the parental sex life and destructiveness. Sometimes, what "the environment offers" are highly idealized forms of perfection and power that become compositional elements in the internal world as ideal objects, both good and bad. The child might feel excluded and persecuted ("the whole world is against me"), or invaded in an absolute and deadly manner, leading to a severe sense of groundlessness and threat. Or, imaginarily, it might form an "us against the world" duo or trio with one of the parents and/or a sibling. In this case, there is always a confusion of identities, and the most grandiose and threatening aspects of people end up bleeding into these same tendencies in the child, creating ideal and violent internal objects. Becoming heir therefore means managing to move beyond these vaunted, willful internal figures by dissolving and modifying them.

As we have seen, Melanie Klein proposes that the development of a new subjectivity depends on the unfolding of the depressive position and the introjection of the good object, especially during the first five years of life, though this needs to be reinforced in a life-long process of self-reconstruction. We will see what these theories – development of the depressive position and introjection of the good object – really mean, as this will help us understand the internal world that needs to be built if we are to be alone in the presence of others.

Working through the depressive position entails separating oneself from that originary symbiosis and all the violent and most Thanatic demands for love that go with it, moderating and eroticizing them so as to preserve the independence of the loved other and the project of consolidation as a new subject. However, there is always the risk of falling towards the polar extremes: either irredeemably fusing with loved-ones and so never being born psychically, or, in order to defend against this kind of psychic death, ignoring people and destroying their value so that they cease to have any significant existence. But then, too, it would be impossible to subjectivize; the living bricks and mortar, which could potentially have become someone, are destroyed in the process.

Early on, Melanie Klein realized that it was essential that we go through a process of mourning for, and resurrection from, those earliest loves, so that we can be born psychically. This mourning and separation present in the depressive position are similar to the development of the Oedipus complex through the castration complex as described by Freud. Ronald Britton, a neo-Kleinian thinker, goes so far as to say: "we resolve the Oedipus complex by working through the depressive position, and the depressive position by working through the Oedipus complex, though neither is ever completed and both need to be worked on with each new life situation". (Britton, 2003, p. 53).

But why does each new life situation and portion of the self require so much mourning in order to be born? We have to slay the "gods" of childhood and the magnificent infant, perfect and absolute alongside the parents in a narcissistic triad. It's a case of abandoning the most absolute need to be loved and the most idealized or denigrated representations of ourselves and our parents and siblings, the other Oedipal characters.

The desire to be everything to someone, maintaining thereby a passional fascination, has to be let go of, so that we can accept a relationship in which our partners have a life and pleasures of their own.

We need to unravel these originary knots. We might say those more narcissistic moments that have to be let slip into the past involve relationships of mutual fascination and dependence, some two-body, others three-body – narcissistic dyads and triads, every bit as intense as they are imprisoning, constituting what we might call the ideal good object. This ideal is magnificent and absolute, but it rapidly becomes threatening and persecutory, as it sets a very high bar of perfection and demand.

The so-called "ideal good object" is the monstrous construction of a dynamism that blends everything that is most passional in our demand for love with all that is most primitive and absolute in the other's demands for love: the result is a reciprocal fascination. Dyads occur when we live the fantasy of plenitude à deux, while the most primitive triad is that which we form with the parental couple – but in this there is always a strong dose of non-differentiation between man and woman, children and parents, sex and tenderness: in other words, confusion between sexual identities and generations. If there can be fusion and a lack of differentiation, there can also be a separation of sex and tenderness, or a desexualized tenderness, because the narcissistic state also gives rise to radical oppositions in which one pole has to annul and repel the other. This description shows us that these "ideal good objects" are jumbled knots of desires and demands for perfection that need to be unravelled if we are to develop a mind of our own.[13]

In contrast with the ideal objects, the good-enough object stems from an experience very different to the unbounded passion, the illusion of being everything that becomes so absolute that it denies the small and humdrum aspects of the experience of loving. The good-enough object corresponds to the unfolding of the Oedipus complex and the depressive position. It is both the origin and the goal of the capacity to be alone. It is the name, indeed, of an experience of pleasure, comfort and safety in the residual presence of a relational dynamism, the memory that, in the beginning, there were two people there – one of whom needed something that the other provided, and for which the former feels grateful. There is a greater differentiation and alliance between masculine and feminine, parental and filial.

The good object is, therefore, a name, with the ability that names possess to transport us someplace else. Thinking about this, I understand much better Lacan's insistence on the paternal metaphor, the "name of the father". The signifier being a father is what transports us to somewhere else, to a symbolic, metaphorizing dimension. The immediate experience is launched towards new potential meanings. What are the functions of the father? To prohibit, regulate, mediate. Protect, furnish a sense of security, provide. Create and distribute the goods we need to live, as in some primitive work of engineering that transports distant water to somewhere close to hand, inventing the means to channel, build, supply.[14] It is not hard to remember the creative displacements of a poem, or an inspired work of fiction, capable of renaming and re-signifying the world of insignificant or paralyzing facts.

The good-enough object is a memorial, a rumor of traversed distances. In its echo, in the distance of being remembered, it is assimilated, giving rise to a new person. A person still to be. Perhaps the greatest virtue of this new person is his future time and desire to change, to become other, and stand apart. In contrast with this, the father of the primitive horde is a burst of arbitrary power and egotism. I imagine the cruel father of the primitive pack as a huge granite block taking up the whole interior of the new subjectivity, as an indissoluble enclave. By building his new "home", the young architect, unable to remove that massive granite rock, has no other choice but to leave it there, filling up all the vital space of the living room, or bedroom. Suffocated, the architect builds the walls of his home around that monolithic obstacle. On the contrary, the good object gives rise to the solid yet subtle foundations of a new subjectivity, but is so infused in them that nobody can see it clearly. The insoluble enclave of the ideal object reveals that, once incorporated, it is unlikely ever to be introjected and integrated into the nascent I, and will remain a model to be imitated or spurned, a voice that judges and condemns, swallowing all the light, as Freud (1917) described in tragic tone: "the shadow of the object fell upon the ego".

In analysis, the analyst becomes receptive to the patient's infantile projections and demands, and allows himself to be tangled up with them so that he might unravel them later through his interpretations and passion to understand how that person functions, both in terms of his or her most profoundly narcissistic needs and desires to form a mind of their own. What are those narcissistic needs? Healthy narcissism is the desire to belong, the desire for union, to be understood, loved, and recognized. It becomes pathological when the subject desires to be fully understood and that the other be fully there, at his disposal, attentive to his every internal movement, whether fears or desires, and ready to soothe them or meet them, tirelessly and without delay. What is the pathological narcissist's greatest aspiration? To find that soulmate that is so utterly transparent that it differs in no way from himself, hides nothing, and keeps nothing to itself. It is, therefore, a demand for equivalence, so that there be no significant difference whatsoever between I and the other. What other? Alterity has to be erased. Either that or this soulmate needs to be like the genie from Aladdin's lamp, to whom my every wish is his command. It is the desire for absolute empathy, complicity, total solidarity from the other, regardless of what I have done or said. It is the movement that leads the patient to appropriate what the analyst has said, immediately making it his own through a process that blurs all differentiation, a desire to be one and the same with the other.

And beyond the most absolute narcissistic demands, what exactly is this desire to have a mind of one's own of which Caper (2005) speaks? It is a desire to separate oneself from the other, to make contact with the solitude that we alone can know, to re-encounter the passion for internal objects. It involves rediscovering the pleasure of looking after oneself and taking responsibility for one's own happiness before demanding it from the world. In other words, it requires stepping outside of our old magical universe. In this it is essential that I see the other as someone separate from myself, and maintain a relationship very different to narcissistic fusion whilst retaining some space for empathy, the possibility of communication, and the healthier aspects of narcissism. The emotions this rouses are complex, and it is painful to see that the other excludes me, that they have a life of their own, which will never be completely transparent or accessible to me; that this other is a thinking person who operates independently of my control and desire. It corresponds to a desire for an autonomy and liberty that exists side-by-side with the narcissistic need to be recognized, belong, and chip away all difference to self.

The analyst endeavors to get to know and name the different desires and demands, to build bridges and connections between them, so that, bringing them into play, the patient can end up drawing meanings from the most fertile springs with which to irrigate the most arid wastelands.

Now, every time, in the nuts-and-bolts of shared existence, someone can forget himself and allow himself to be at least partially forgotten by the other, he becomes, through that, something nourishingly assimilable. When we can be alone in another's presence, the same process of conjunctions and disjunctions, deaths and rebirths described above will be underway or in the process of being resumed.

It is the hard art of learning to treat others, and be treated by others, like a dog asleep on the rug. And that is important if we are to fight the greater temptation of one day wanting to be everything that a dog actually thinks we are.

Notes

1 The Martin Scorcese film *Shutter Island* was released in 2010.
2 Total war is defined as any "war which is unrestricted in terms of the resources or personnel employed, the territory or nations involved, or the objectives pursued; esp. war in which civilians are perceived as combatants and therefore as legitimate targets" (*Oxford English Dictionary*).
3 S. Freud, Draft N.
4 Film based on the Dennis Lehane novel Patient 67, reissued under the title *Shutter Island*. Scorcese has always been interested in the theme of insanity, which he explored in such films as Taxi Driver, Raging Bull, and Cape Fear. Other films that explore the theme are The King of Comedy, After Hours, Goodfellas, and Cassino.
5 Originally recorded by Dinah Washington, "Bitter Earth" can be heard at link: www.youtube.com/watch?v=f9zAUZfDV-w. It's super-blue, very soul, a gorgeous black lament. At this second link, Dinah sings the song to musical backing by Max Richter: www.youtube.com/watch?v=8rluU6BGpKw. The full lyrics are as follows: This bitter earth, What fruit it bears, What good is love, That no one shares, And what if my life is like the dust That hides the glow of a rose, What good am I, Heaven only knows, This bitter Earth Can be so cold, Today you're young, Too soon you are old, But while a voice Within me cries, I'm sure someone May answer my call, And this bitter earth May not be so bitter after all.
6 First published in PULSIONAL – Revista de Psicanálise, São Paulo, years 14 and 15, n. 152/153, p. 70–81, 2001.
7 Text originally published in Cadernos de Psicanálise – Sociedade de Psicanálise da Cidade do Rio de Janeiro v.23, n.26, Rio de Janeiro, 2007. Debate theme – SOLIDÃO. p. 35–51. Original title: "Trate-me como um cachorro. Ou assim que for possível".
8 In Kleinian terms, this entails a safe introjection of the good object, which, as we shall see further on, is very different to the presence of the ideal object, an insoluble enclave of the unintrojectable and unassimilable.
9 Cf. "The Intuition of the Negative in Playing and Reality", by André Green, 1997.
10 The poem "Casamento" is from the book *Terra de Santa Cruz*.
11 Freud (1905) described a universal childhood fantasy of the parents in a sadomasochistic sexual relation.
12 Melanie Klein (1928), on the other hand, named this kind of fantasy "the combined-parent figure", which becomes far more threatening and persecutory, as they "gang up" on the child, who can no longer count on the protection of either parent in moments of aggression, and is so left at the mercy of combined parental violence. The child feels as though everyone is against him.

13 Cf. "Having a Mind of One's Own", by Robert Caper. In: Caper, R. Having a Mind of One's Own: A Psychoanalytic View of Self and Object. Routledge, 1998.
14 There's a film called *The Painted Veil*, which is set in rural China, where a cholera epidemic has killed much of the population and almost all the water is contaminated. But then along comes a young English doctor, who tries to fight the epidemic by designing a simple system using lengths of bamboo to channel uncontaminated water to the village.

References

Bollas, C. (1999). *The mistery of things*. London; New York: Routledge.
Britton, R. (1998). *Belief and imagination: Explorations in psychoanalysis*. London; New York: Routledge.
Bruneteau, B. (2005). *Le siècle des génocides. Violences, massacres et processus génocidaires de l'Arménie au Rwanda*. Paris: Armand Colin. (Translation: The Century of Genocides).
Caper, R. A. (2005). *A mind of one's own – A psychoanalytic view of self and object*. London: Routledge.
Cintra, E. M. U. (2006). Trate-me como um cachorro. *Cadernos de Psicanálise*, v. 22, pp. 35–51.
Cintra, E. M. U. (2001). Hamlet e a melancolia. Revista Latinoamericana de Psicopatologia Fundamentalimage, São Paulo, v. 4, n.4, pp. 30–42. (Translation: Hamlet and the melancholia).
Cintra, E. M. U. (2001). Luto e melancolia: uma reflexão sobre purificar e o destruir. Free translation: "Mourning and Melancholia: A Reflection on Purifying and Destroying". *Alter Revista de Estudos Psicanalíticos*, v. 29, n. 1, pp. 23–40.
Freud, S. (1905/2024). Three essays. In: *The revised standard edition of the complete psychological works of Sigmund Freud*. Translated by James Strachey and revised by Mark Solms. London: Rowman and Littlefield.
Freud, S. (1910/2024). Psychoanalytic notes on an autobiographical account of a case of paranoia (dementia paranoides). In: *The revised standard edition of the complete psychological works of Sigmund Freud*. Translated by James Strachey and revised by Mark Solms. London: Rowman and Littlefield.
Freud, S. (1914/2024). On narcissism: An introduction. In: *The revised standard edition of the complete psychological works of Sigmund Freud*. Translated by James Strachey and revised by Mark Solms. London: Rowman and Littlefield.
Freud, S. (1916/2024). Some character-types met with in psycho-analytic work. In: *The revised standard edition of the complete psychological works of Sigmund Freud*. Translated by James Strachey and revised by Mark Solms. London: Rowman and Littlefield.
Freud, S. (1917/2024). Mourning and melancholia. In: *The revised standard edition of the complete psychological works of Sigmund Freud*. Translated by James Strachey and revised by Mark Solms. London: Rowman and Littlefield.
Freud, S. (1925/2024). Denial. In: *The revised standard edition of the complete psychological works of Sigmund Freud*. Translated by James Strachey and revised by Mark Solms. London: Rowman and Littlefield.
Freud, S. (1937/2024). Analysis terminable and interminable. In: *The revised standard edition of the complete psychological works of Sigmund Freud*. Translated by James Strachey and revised by Mark Solms. London: Rowman and Littlefield.

Green, A. (1993). *Le travail du négatif*. Paris: Minuit. (translation: The work of the negative).

Green, A. (1997/1999). The Intuition of the negative in playing and reality. In: Kohon, G. (org.) *The dead mother*. Londres: Routledge.

Guimarães Rosa, J. (1962). *Primeiras estórias*. Rio de Janeiro: Livraria José Olympio Editora. (Translation: The third bank of the river and other stories).

Karl, A. (1924/1979). The influence of oral erotism on character formation. In: *Selected papers on psycho-analysis*. New York: Brunner/Mazel.

Klein, M. (1928/1960). Early stages of the Oedipus conflict and of super-ego formation. In: *The psychoanalysis of children*. New York: Grove Press.

Klein, M. (1935/1975). A contribution to the psychogenesis of manic-depressive states. In: *Love, guilt and reparation other works*. New York: Dell Publishing Co.

Klein, M. (1940/1975). Mourning and it relation to manic-depressive states. In: *Love, guilt and reparation and other works*. New York: Dell Publishing Co.

Kristeva, J. (1999). *Le génie féminin: la vie, la folie, les mots: Hannah Arendt, Melanie Klein, Colette*. Paris: Fayard. (Translation: Female Genius: life, madness, words – Hannah Arendt, Melanie Klein, Colette; a Trilogy).

Levinas, E. (1971). *Totalité et Infini – essai sur l'exteririté*. Paris: Le Livre de Poche. (Translation: Totality and infinity: an essay on exteriority).

Pinto, J. N. (2001). *Confissões de Bin Laden*. O Estado de São Paulo, p. A2. Available in https://acervo.estadao.com.br/pagina/#!/20011010-39439-nac-2-opi-a2-not. Accessed in 11/25/2024.

Pontalis, J-B. (1988/1991*). Perder de vista. Da fantasia de recuperação do objeto perdido*. (Trad. Vera Ribeiro). Rio de Janeiro: Jorge Zahar Editor. (Translation: Losing sight).

Prado, A. (1971/1991) Terra de Santa Cruz. In: *Poesia Reunida*. São Paulo: Siciliano. (Translation: Land of Santa Cruz. In: Selected Poems).

Rilke, R. M. (1939). *Duino elegies*. New York: W. W. Norton & Company.

Semelin, J. (2009). *Purificar e destruir*. (Trad. Jorge Bastos). Rio de Janeiro: Difel. (Translation: Purify and destroy: the political uses of massacre and genocide).

Shakespeare, W. (1603/2003). *Hamlet*. London: Penguin Classics.

Winnicott, D. W. (1958/1990). The capacity to be alone. In: *Maturational processes and the facilitating environment*. London; New York: Karnac.

Winnicott, D. W. (1963/1990). The development of the capacity for concern. In: *Maturational processes and the facilitating environment*. London; New York: Karnac.

Film references

Shutter Island. (2010). Directed by Martin Scorsese; screenplay by Laeta Kalogridis. Paramount Pictures.

The Painted Veil. (2006). Directed by John Curran; screenplay by Ronald Harwood. Warner Bros.

Song reference

Veloso, C. (1984). A terceira margem do rio. On Velô. Philips Records. (Translation: the third bank of the river).

Appendix A
Some works about Melanie Klein

Some works on Melanie Klein

Dictionary of Kleinian Thought. Robert Douglas Hinshelwood. Jason Aronson Inc, 1984.

Melanie Klein and beyond: A bibliography of primary and secondary sources. Harry Karnac, 2009.

The new dictionary of kleinian thought. Elizabeth Bott Spillius, Jane Milton, Penelope Garvey, Cyril Couve and Deborah Steiner. London & NY Routledge, 2011.

Biographies of Melanie Klein

Melanie Klein: Her world and her work. Phyllis Grosskurth. The Harvard University Press, 1986.

Studies of the work of Melanie Klein

Melanie Klein: First discoveries and first system 1919-1932: v. 1. Jean-Michel Petot. International Universities Press Inc, 1990.

Melanie Klein: The ego and the good object, 1932-1960: vol.2. Petot, Jean-Michel. . International Universities Press Inc, 1991.

Significant works based on the thought of Melanie Klein

Belief and imagination. Explorations in psychoanalysis. Ronald Britton. Routledge, 1998.

".... But at the same time and on another level..." Psychoanalytic theory and technique in the Kleinian/Bionian Mode. Vol 1.e Vol. 2. Clinical applications in the kleinian/bionian mode. James S. Grotstein. London: Karnac, 2009.

Clinical Klein: From theory to practice. Robert D. Hinshelwood. Basic Books, 1994.

Clinical Lectures on Klein and Bion. Elizabeth Bott Spillius; Robin Anderson (Ed.). Routledge, 1992.

Contemporary object relations in Los Angeles: Building on the work of the London Kleinians. Jennifer Langham (Ed). Phoenix Publishing House, 2023.

Dream, phantasy and art. Hannah Segal. Routledge, 1990.

Encounters with Melanie Klein: Selected papers of Elizabeth Spillius. Elizabeth Spillius; Dana Birksted-Breen; Priscilla Roth; Richard Rusbridger. London & Nova York: Routledge, 2007.

Envy and gratitude revisited. Priscilla Roth and Alessandra Lemma (Eds). R. Horácio Etchegoyen (forward). London: Karnac, 2008.

Essential Readings from the Melanie Klein archive: Original papers and critical Reflections. Jane Milton. Routledge, 2020.

Freud and beyond: A history of modern psychoanalytic thought. Stephen A. Mitchell; Margaret J. Black. Basic Books, 1995.

From anthropology to psychoanalysis. In Encounters with Melanie Klein: Selected papers of Elizabeth Spillius. Elizabeth Spillius; Dana Birksted-Breen; Priscilla Roth; Richard Rusbridger. London & Nova York: Routledge, 2007.

Guilt and depression. León Gringberg; Christine Trollope. Karnac Books, 1992.

In pursuit of psychic change: The Betty Joseph workshop. Dana Birksted-Breen; Edith Hargreaves; Arturo Varchevker. Brunner Routledge, 2004.

Lectures on technique by Melanie Klein. John Steiner (Ed). London and New York: Routledge, 2017.

Melanie Klein & critical social theory. An account of politics, art and reason based on her psychoanalytic theory. C. Fred Alford. Yale: Yale University Press, 1989.

Melanie Klein: A contemporary introduction. Penelope Garvey. Routledge, 2023.

Melanie Klein: From theory to reality. Otto Weininger. Karnac Books, 1992.

Melanie Klein's narrative of an adult analysis. Christine English. 2023. Routledge, 2023.

Melanie Klein revisited: Pioneer and revolutionary in the psychoanalysis of young children. Susan Sherwin-White. Karnac, 2017.

Melanie Klein: The basics. Robert D. Hinshelwood and Tomasz Fortuna. Routledge, 2017.

Melanie Klein today. Elizabeth Bott Spillius et al. London: Routledge, 1988.

A mind of one's own. A kleinian view of self and object. Robert Caper. Routledge, 1999.

Portrait of a life: Melanie Klein and the artists. Roger Amos. Phoenix, 2019.

Projective identification and psychotherapeutic technique. Thomas Ogden. New York: Jason Aronson, 1982.

Projective identification. The fate of a concept. Elizabeth Spillius and Edna O'Shaughnessy. Londres & Nova York: Routledge, 2012.

Projective identification in the clinical setting: The kleinian interpretation. Robert Waska. Brunner Routledge, 2004.

Psychic equilibrium and psychic change: Selected papers of Betty Joseph. Betty Joseph, Michael Feldman, Elizabeth Bott Spillius. Londres & Nova York: Routledge, 1989.

Psychic retreats: Pathological organizations in psychotic, neurotic and border-line patients. John Steiner. Londres & Nova York: Routledge, 1993.

Psychoanalysis and anxiety: From knowing to being. Chris Mawson. Routledge, 2019.

Psychoanalysis, literature and war: Papers 1972-1995. Hannah Segal. Routledge, 1997.

Psychoanalytic psychotherapy in the kleinian tradition. Stanley Ruszczynski; Sue Johnson. Karnac Books, 1999.

Reading Klein. Margaret Rustin e Michael Rustin. London & N.Y: Routledge, 2017.

Reading Melanie Klein. Lyndsey Stonebridge and John Phillips (Eds). London and New York: Routledge, 1998.

Real people, real problems, real solutions: The kleinian psychoanalytic approach with difficult patients. Robert Waska. Brunner Routledge, 2005.

Selected Melanie Klein. Juliet Mitchell. London: Simon & Schuster, 1987.

Splitting and projective identification. James Grotstein. Jason Aronson, 1981.

Subjects of Analysis. Thomas Ogden. Jason Aronson, 1994.

Suffering insanity: Psychoanalytic essays on psychosis. Robert D. Hinshelwood. Brunner Routledge, 2004.

The bounds of reason: Habermas, Lyotard and Melanie Klein on rationality. Emilia Steuerman. Routledge, 1999.

The clinical paradigms of Melanie Klein and Donald Winnicott: Comparisons and dialogues. Jan Abram and Robert D. Hinshelwood. Routledge, 2018.

The contemporary kleinians of London. Schafer, R. Madison: International University Press, 1997.

The Freud-Klein controversies 1941-1945. Pearl King & Riccardo Steiner. Routledge, 1991.

The good society and the inner world – Psychoanalysis, politics and culture. Michael Rustin. London: Verso, 1991.

The Klein tradition: Lines of development – Evolution of theory and practice over the decades. Penelope Garvey and Kay Long. Routledge, 2018.

The matrix of the mind. Object Relations and the Psychoanalytic Dialogue. Thomas H. Ogden. Jason Aronson Inc, 1986

The Oedipus complex today: Clinical implications. Ronald Britton; Michael Feldman; Edna O'Shaughnessy; John Steiner. Karnac Books, 1989.

Trauma, guilt and reparation: The path from impasse to development. Heinz Weiss. Routledge, 2019.

What evil means to us. C. Fred Alford. Cornell. University Press, 1997.

Yesterday, today and tomorrow. Hanna Segal. London & NY: Routledge, 2007.

Reading Klein. Margaret and Michael Rustin. London & NY: Routledge, 2017.

Some reference articles

Affects in Melanie Klein. By Rusbridger, Richard. International Journal of Psychoanalysis, v. 93, n. 1, February, 2012.

A new reading of the origins of object-relations theory. By Thomas H. Ogden. The International Journal of Psychoanalysis v. *83*, n. 4, pp. 767–782, 2002. https://doi.org/10.1516/LX9C-R1P9-F1BV-2L96

The ego according to Klein: Return to Freud and beyond. By Blass, Rachel B. International Journal of Psychoanalysis, v. 93, n. 1, February 2012.

The elusive concept of 'internal objects' (1934–1943). Its role in the formation of the Klein Group. By Robert D. Hinshelwood. International Journal of Psychoanalysis. v. 78, n.5, pp. 877–897, 1997

Some technical implications of Klein's concept of "premature ego development". By Mitrani, Judith L. International Journal of Psychoanalysis, v. 88, August 2007.

Classics of the Kleinian thought

Developments in Psychoanalysis. Klein, M.; Heimann, P.; Isaacs, S. & Riviere, J. London: the Hogarth Press, 1952.

Introduction to the work of Melanie Klein. Segal, H. London: The Hogarth Press, 1973.

New direction in psycho- analysis. Part I and II. Klein, M.; Heimann, P. & Money-Kyrle, R. London: Tavistock Publications, 1955/1969.

Other books on the thought of Klein, Bion, and Winnicott

On Bion

A beam of intense darkness. Wilfred Bion's Legacy on Psychoanalysis. James Grotstein. Karnac Books, 2007.

The clinical thinking of Wilfred Bion. Joan Neville Symington. Routledge, 1996.

Attacks on linking revisited: A new look at Bion's Classic Work. Catalina Bronstein and Elizabeth O'Shaughnessy (Eds.). Karnac, 2007.

Bion and thoughts too deep for words: Psychoanalysis, suggestion, and the language of the unconscious. Caper, R. Routledge, 2020.

Bion: An introduction. Nicola Abel-Hirsch. Phoenix Publishing House, 2023.

Bion in Buenos Aires: Seminars, case presentation and supervision. Joseph Aguayo, Lia Pistiner de Cortinas and Agnes Regeczkey, A. (Eds.). Karnac, 2017.

Bion: 365 quotes. Nicola Abel-Hirsch. Routledge, 2019.

Who is the Dreamer who Dreams the Dream and who is the Dreamer who Understands It—A Psychoanalytic Inquiry Into the Ultimate Nature of Being. James Grotstein. *Contemporary Psychoanalysis*. 1979, *(15)*, 110–169.

On Meltzer

The Kleinian development: This series is divided into three parts, each focusing on a key figure in psychoanalysis:

- *Part 1: Freud's clinical development – Method–data–theory*: Examines Sigmund Freud's clinical development.
- *Part 2: Richard week-by-week – Melanie Klein's 'Narrative of a child analysis'*: Provides an in-depth analysis of Klein's work, particularly her 'Narrative of a Child Analysis'.
- *Part 3: The clinical significance of the work of Bion*: focuses on Wilfred Bion's contributions.

The Apprehension of beauty: The role of Aesthetic conflict in development, Art, and violence: Co-authored with Meg Harris Williams, this book explores the aesthetic dimensions of psychoanalytic theory, building upon Klein's ideas.

The claustrum: An investigation of claustrophobic phenomena: In this work, Meltzer examines claustrophobic phenomena through a Kleinian lens, expanding on concepts related to projective identification and internal objects.

Meltzer in Paris. Jacques Touze (Ed.). Harris Meltzer Trust, 2017.

Sincerity and other works: Collected papers of Donald Meltzer. Donald Meltzer; Alberto Hahn. Karnac Books, 1994.

On Winnicott

Reading Winnicott. Dana Birksted-Breen; Lesley Caldwell; Angela Joyce. Londres & Nova York: Routledge, 2011.

The goals of psychoanalysis: Identification, identity, and supervision. León Gringberg. Karnac Books, 1990.

Appendix B
A brief biography of Melanie Klein

1882 Melanie Reizes is born in Vienna on March 30th. She was the daughter of Moriz Reizes and Libussa Deustsch, and the youngest of four siblings: Emilie, Emanuel, Sidonie, and Melanie. Her father was a doctor and dentist, as well as an orthodox Jew. Her mother was 24 years younger than her father, and this was his second marriage. When Klein was four years old, she lost her sister Sidonie. She lost her father when she was 18 years old and at 20, she lost her dear brother Emanuel. These early experiences of grief marked Klein's life and thought.

1903 Melanie marries Arthur Klein. He was the best friend of her brother Emanuel, who had recently passed away. Klein's marriage hindered her from becoming a doctor like her father.

1904 Her daughter Melitta Klein is born. Arthur Klein's profession as an engineer required him to frequently relocate, which Melanie would try to keep up with. She took care of Melitta until she was 7 months old. After that, she left her daughter in the care of her mother and caretakers.

1907 Her son Hans is born. Klein experiences intense depressive symptoms after the birth of her son. Libussa moves in with the Klein family to help take care of the children. Feelings of rivalry are intensely present between Melanie and Libussa and, in the future, between Melanie and Melitta.

1910 The family moves to Budapest, where Melanie Klein becomes familiar with Freud's work through the book *The interpretation of dreams*.

1913 Ferenczi establishes the Hungarian Psychoanalysis Society.

1914 Birth of Erich Klein. A few months later, Libussa passes away. Arthur goes to war. Melanie starts analysis with Sándor Ferenczi, which continues throughout World War I.

1918 The 5th International Psychoanalytic Congress is held in Budapest, presided over by Ferenczi.

1919 Klein presents her first article and becomes a member of the Hungarian Psychoanalytic Society. Ernest Jones, a former analysand of Ferenczi, founds the British Psychoanalytical Society. Klein finds in psychoanalysis a possibility to fulfill her intellectual ambitions.

1920 During the 6th International Psychoanalytic Congress, in The Hague, Klein meets Karl Abraham, who would later become her analyst and supporter.

1921 Klein moves to Berlin where she starts her clinical practice for analysis of adults and children. Melitta engages in Medical School in Berlin.

1922 Klein becomes an Associate Member of the Berlin Psychoanalytic Society. Abraham, like Ferenczi, encourages her to offer psychoanalytic treatment for children. Melanie and Arthur Klein get divorced.

1924 Foundation of the British Psycho-Analytic Institute. Klein begins analysis with Karl Abraham. In Salzburg, during the 8th International Psychoanalytic Congress, she presents a paper on the technique of child analysis. Later it becomes the second chapter of the book "*The Psycho-Analysis of Children*".

1925 After being invited by Ernest Jones, the future biographer of Freud, Klein presents a series of lectures in London. Karl Abraham passes away at the age of 48, which interrupts Klein's second analysis. Both her analysts died prematurely.

1926 Klein moves to London. She becomes the analyst of Ernest Jones' children. She quickly becomes well known as a child analyst of children.

1927 Klein is elected as a member of the British Psychoanalytical Society.

1928 Melitta meets Walter Schmideberg, a member of the Berlin Psychoanalytic Society and also her future husband.

1932 Klein's first book "*The Psycho-Analysis of Children*" is published in English and German. Klein is then a training analyst.

1933 Melitta, which by then uses her married name Schmideberg, is elected as a member of the British Psychoanalytic Society. She becomes a public and fierce opponent of Klein.

1934 Melanie's son Hans dies while mountain climbing. In the process of such difficult grief, she writes the article "*A Contribution to the Psychogenesis of Manic-Depressive States*", published in 1935.

1937 The book "*Love, Guilt and Reparation*" is published.

1939 Klein moves to Cambridge to escape the bombings in London. Freud dies on September 23rd.

1941 Klein returns to London. The British Psychoanalytical Society promotes debates regarding the changes introduced by Klein into Freudian theory. These would be later known as "*The Freud–Klein Controversies*".

1941–1945 The "*Freud–Klein Controversies*" period. Anna Freud and Melanie Klein diverge on several points, especially on a child's capacity to establish transference and its elaboration. As a result of these discussions, a book with the same name is published. Additionally, three groups were formed within the British Psychoanalytical Society: the Freudians, the Kleinians and the independent group, of which Winnicott was a member.

1945 Melitta moves to the United States; mother and daughter never reconciled. The bond between Klein, her third son Erich and her grandchildren remained until the end of her life, bringing her feelings of fulfillment.

1946 Klein publishes the article *"Notes on some schizoid mechanism"*, in which she formulates the concept of projective identification.

1952 A Special Edition of the *International Journal of Psychoanalysis* is published as a tribute to Melanie Klein's 70th birthday. The book *"Developments in Psychoanalysis"* is published by Klein, Paula Heimann, Susan Isaacs, and Joan Riviere.

1955 Foundation of the Melanie Klein Trust. Current website: www.melanie-klein-trust.org.uk. The book *"New Directions in Psychoanalysis: The Significance of Infant Conflict in the Pattern of Adult Behaviour"* is published, edited by Klein, Money-Kyrle, and Heimann.

1957 The book *Envy and Gratitude* is published. Just when nothing new was expected from Klein, she surprises the psychoanalytic community with the publication of this book, which becomes the subject of heated discussions.

1958 Ernest Jones, her main supporter, dies.

1960 Melanie Klein passed away in London on September 22nd at the age of 78, following a battle with cancer. Her legacy endures in contemporary psychoanalysis, where her groundbreaking contributions continue to inspire. Over time, her work has been widely recognized for its brilliance, reaffirming her status as a psychoanalyst ahead of her era.

1961 The book *"Narrative of the Analysis of a Child"* is published posthumously. She was working on it just days before her death. It consists of 93 sessions with a ten-year-old boy during her time as a refugee in Cambridge.

Index

For Product Safety Concerns and Information please contact our EU
representative GPSR@taylorandfrancis.com
Taylor & Francis Verlag GmbH, Kaufingerstraße 24, 80331 München, Germany